The Stroke Survival Guide

Mark Greener spent a decade in biomedical research before joining *MIMS Magazine* for GPs in 1989. Since then he has written on health and biology for magazines worldwide for patients, healthcare professionals and scientists. He is the author of 15 other books, including *The Heart Attack Survival Guide* (2012), *The Holistic Health Handbook* (2013) and *Coping with Thyroid Disease* (2014), all for Sheldon Press. Mark lives with his wife, three children and two cats in a Cambridgeshire village.

Overcoming Common Problems Series

Selected titles

A full list of titles is available from Sheldon Press,
36 Causton Street, London SW1P 4ST and on our website at
www.sheldonpress.co.uk

Breast Cancer: Your treatment choices
Dr Terry Priestman

**Chronic Fatigue Syndrome: What you need
to know about CFS/ME**
Dr Megan A. Arroll

Cider Vinegar
Margaret Hills

**Coping Successfully with Chronic Illness:
Your healing plan**
Neville Shone

Coping Successfully with Hiatus Hernia
Dr Tom Smith

Coping with Difficult Families
Dr Jane McGregor and Tim McGregor

Coping with Epilepsy
Dr Pamela Crawford and Fiona Marshall

Coping with Guilt
Dr Windy Dryden

Coping with Liver Disease
Mark Greener

Coping with Memory Problems
Dr Sallie Baxendale

Coping with Obsessive Compulsive Disorder
Professor Kevin Gournay, Rachel Piper
and Professor Paul Rogers

**Coping with the Psychological Effects
of Illness**
Dr Fran Smith, Dr Carina Eriksen
and Professor Robert Bor

Coping with Schizophrenia
Professor Kevin Gournay and Debbie Robson

Coping with Thyroid Disease
Mark Greener

Depressive Illness: The curse of the strong
Dr Tim Cantopher

**The Empathy Trap: Understanding
antisocial personalities**
Dr Jane McGregor and Tim McGregor

**Epilepsy: Complementary and
alternative treatments**
Dr Sallie Baxendale

The Fibromyalgia Healing Diet
Christine Craggs-Hinton

Fibromyalgia: Your treatment guide
Christine Craggs-Hinton

Hay Fever: How to beat it
Dr Paul Carson

Helping Elderly Relatives
Jill Eckersley

The Holistic Health Handbook
Mark Greener

How to Eat Well When You Have Cancer
Jane Freeman

How to Stop Worrying
Dr Frank Tallis

**Invisible Illness: Coping with
misunderstood conditions**
Dr Megan A. Arroll and Professor
Christine P. Dancey

Living with Complicated Grief
Professor Craig A. White

Living with Fibromyalgia
Christine Craggs-Hinton

Living with Hearing Loss
Dr Don McFerran, Lucy Handscomb
and Dr Cherilee Rutherford

Living with IBS
Nuno Ferreira and David T. Gillanders

Overcoming Fear: With mindfulness
Deborah Ward

Overcoming Stress
Professor Robert Bor, Dr Carina Eriksen
and Dr Sara Chaudry

Overcoming Worry and Anxiety
Dr Jerry Kennard

**Physical Intelligence: How to take charge
of your weight**
Dr Tom Smith

The Self-Esteem Journal
Alison Waines

The Stroke Survival Guide
Mark Greener

Ten Steps to Positive Living
Dr Windy Dryden

Treating Arthritis: The drug-free way
Margaret Hills and Christine Horner

Treating Arthritis: The supplements guide
Julia Davies

**Understanding Yourself and Others: Practical
ideas from the world of coaching**
Bob Thomson

**When Someone You Love Has Depression:
A handbook for family and friends**
Barbara Baker

Overcoming Common Problems

The Stroke Survival Guide

MARK GREENER

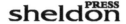

To Rose, Yasmin, Rory and Ophelia with love

First published in Great Britain in 2015

Sheldon Press
36 Causton Street
London SW1P 4ST
www.sheldonpress.co.uk

British Library Cataloguing-in-Publication Data
A catalogue record for this book is available from the British Library

ISBN 978–1–84709–309–7
eBook ISBN 978–1–84709–310–3

Typeset by Fakenham Prepress Solutions, Fakenham, Norfolk NR21 8NN
First printed in Great Britain by Ashford Colour Press
Subsequently digitally reprinted in Great Britain

eBook by Fakenham Prepress Solutions, Fakenham, Norfolk NR21 8NN

Produced on paper from sustainable forests

Contents

Note to the reader

This is not a medical book and is not intended to replace advice from your doctor or another health professional. Consult your pharmacist, nurse or doctor if you believe you have any of the symptoms described, and if you think you might need medical help.

Introduction

By the time you have read this introduction, someone, some-where in the UK will probably have suffered a stroke. The Stroke Association says that about 152,000 people suffer a stroke each year – that's about one person every five minutes. One stroke in five is fatal, which made strokes the fourth most common cause of death in the UK during 2010. Only cancer, heart disease and respiratory (lung) diseases killed more people. Indeed, strokes kill about one in 14 men and one in ten women.

Despite these bleak figures, the chances of surviving a stroke are better than ever. The Health Survey for England suggests that deaths from stroke declined by 42 per cent between 2003 and 2011.[1] The UK is now home to about 1.1 million stroke survivors – that's approximately twice the population of Manchester. However, modern treatments mean that while more people recover more fully after a stroke, more people survive with more severe disabilities than in the past.

Stroke's physical, mental and emotional legacy varies from person to person. However, as a rule, strokes leave half the survivors permanently, and sometimes severely, disabled. For instance, many survivors are unable to perform tasks most of us take for granted – such as walking, bathing, dressing, eating and using the toilet – at least for a while after their stroke.

The NHS's stroke rehabilitation teams use techniques tailored to a person's needs, goals and circumstances to ensure that each sur-vivor recovers his or her maximum possible physical, functional, psychological and social function within the limits imposed by any disability.[2] Nevertheless, your recovery depends on your com-mitment and that of your partner or other carers. You will need, for example, to practise regularly the exercises suggested by the stroke team. You will need to learn to live within any disability and, perhaps, to adapt to changes in your relationships with partner, family and friends. In addition, you will need to make lifestyle changes to reduce the risk of another stroke.

While many people recover fully after a stroke, do not underesti-mate the challenges. Sometimes a stroke leaves hidden disabilities, such as problems with memory, thinking and concentration, depression and anxiety, and personality changes. Healthcare professionals know about these changes. However, the 'sympathy', help and support that stroke survivors and their carers receive is often much less for these hidden problems than for physical disabilities. Yet the hidden problems can be just as upsetting, just as difficult to live with, just as distressing as physical disabilities.

In addition, many people – including relatives themselves – ignore carers' needs: a stroke can turn a family's life upside down and may dramatically alter relationships between partners or across the generations. Not surprisingly, carers are prone to stress, anxiety and depression and receive, tragically, very little support. For instance, a lack of information is a major problem for people with stroke and their families.[3] So, I hope that spouses, family members and other carers gain as much from this book as survivors. I wrote the book for you all. Recovering from stroke is a partnership between families, professionals and survivors.

Preventing another stroke

A stroke usually means fundamentally changing your lifestyle, not just to live with any disability, but also to prevent another stroke. Once you survive a stroke – even a 'mini-stroke', also called a transient ischaemic attack (TIA) – you are much more likely to suffer another, even if you recover fully in between. For example, 11 per cent of people have another stroke within a year of their first stroke. Around 26 per cent have another stroke within five years and 39 per cent have another one within ten years.[4] Stroke survivors carry a similar risk of developing other cardiovascular (heart and blood vessel) diseases, such as a heart attack.[5]

In other words, stroke survivorship is not just about living as full a life as possible; it is also about avoiding another stroke. Yet, only 23 per cent of people who survived a TIA told a Stroke Association survey published as *Not just a funny turn* (available at <http://www.stroke.org.uk/tia-briefing>) that healthcare professionals did not give information or advice about the lifestyle changes that prevent a full-blown stroke.

In addition, a type of irregular heartbeat called atrial fibrillation (see page 35) causes around 12,500 strokes each year, according to the

National Institute for Health and Clinical Excellence (NICE). Drugs called anticoagulants (which prevent blood clots) protect against stroke in these vulnerable people. However, NICE notes that only 45 per cent of eligible people currently receive anticoagulants. NICE estimates that effective detection and using anticoagulants could avoid around 7,000 strokes and 2,000 premature deaths every year.

In other words, you need to take responsibility for your health and well-being. As the risk of recurrence is highest in the days and weeks immediately after the stroke or TIA, you should start as soon as possible and stick to a healthy lifestyle for the rest of your life.[5] Even simple changes can make a dramatic difference. For instance, combining medicines and lifestyle changes can reduce a survivor's risk of cardiovascular diseases – such as a further stroke or heart attack – by 80 per cent over 5 years.[6]

However, if this book has a single message, it's that you, your carers, your family, friends and colleagues need to know the signs that suggest that you may have suffered a TIA or stroke and get help as soon as possible. The more quickly you are treated, the better your chances of recovery. Rapid treatment may even save your life. As geriatrician Richard Lindley notes 'Time is brain'.[7]

Time to act fast

About 95 per cent of people experience their first symptoms of a stroke outside hospital.[5] So, you *must* seek medical attention as soon as you or someone around you develops one or more symptoms that might indicate a stroke. The sooner you act the better the chances of a full recovery. Call 999 or go to the local accident and emergency department if you or someone around you experiences any of the following:[8]

- Weakness or numbness in the face, arm or leg – Can the person smile? Has his or her eye or mouth dropped? Can he or she raise both arms?[7]
- Loss or slurring of speech – Can the person speak clearly and understand what you say?[7]
- Loss or blurring of vision
- A sensation of motion (vertigo)
- Difficulty with balance
- Unusual, sudden or severe headache.

Nevertheless, even after rapid treatment, recovering from a stroke can take a long time and seem slow, frustrating and even, from time to time, futile. While stroke teams are caring, skilled and compassionate, they do not have the time or resources to do everything possible for every patient immediately. That might be one reason why, according to the UK guidelines for stroke care, nearly half of survivors still have unmet needs between one and five years after their stroke.[5]

In addition, stroke can damage the survivor's ability to remember, understand and communicate. This makes accessing the help that the survivor needs even more difficult. I hope carers will read the book and I suggest that they should be around when the survivor receives instructions from the rehabilitation team or other health-care professionals: everyone needs to know what he or she needs to do and why. After all, even healthy people can find remembering everything a doctor tells them difficult.

This book looks at the causes and risk factors for stroke. It considers prevention, treatment and rehabilitation. And we shall see why carers need to help themselves to help the stroke survivor. A stroke is devastating for the survivor and, often, for the partner, family and friends. But I hope this book helps you not just survive, but also thrive, after a stroke.

A word to the wise

This book does not replace advice from doctors, nurses, therapists or pharmacists who tailor suggestions, support and treatment to your circumstances. Always see a doctor if you feel unwell, if you think that your signs, symptoms or disability are getting worse or if you are worried that you have symptoms that could indicate a stroke, another form of cardiovascular disease or that you have developed side effects.

While I have included numerous references from medical and scientific studies, it has been impossible to cite all those I used. (Apologies to anyone whose work I have missed.) The articles referenced illustrate some important points and themes, and are a starting point if you want to know more. Some papers may seem rather erudite if you do not have a medical or biological background. Do not let this put you off: they are usually understandable if you do some background reading and ask questions.

You can find a summary of each article by entering its title or other details here: <www.ncbi.nlm.nih.gov/pubmed/citmatch>. Some full papers are available free online, while a growing number of publishers offer patients relatively cheap access. Larger libraries might stock or allow you to access some better-known medical journals. The better informed you are, the better you will be able to tackle the problems following a stroke.

1

Your remarkable brain

Your brain is the most remarkable organ in your body. After all, the brain is, the American writer Ambrose Bierce quipped, the 'apparatus with which we think that we think'. This soft blob – writers compare its consistency to a jelly, soft tofu or warm butter – is responsible for your intelligence, emotions and personality.

In 1848, for example, an explosion sent an iron rod weighing six kilograms (13 pounds) through the head of Phineas Gage, a 25-year-old rail worker. Remarkably, Gage survived. However, Gage – previously patient, responsible and mild-mannered – became impulsive and inconsistent and would swear at the slightest provocation.[9]

Gage offers an extreme example of how a brain injury can change personality. Similarly, strokes can damage the brain and, sometimes, change the survivor's personality. A person who was 'happy-go-lucky' before the stroke may become depressed. A person who was responsible or conservative may become impulsive or behave inappropriately. A person who was careful and calm may become hurried and anxious.[10]

Strokes occur when the blood supply to the brain becomes blocked. The cells supplied by that part of the brain die because they do not have sufficient oxygen and nutrients. The effects depend on the part of the brain damaged:

- Damage to a part of the brain that controls movement can cause one or more 'motor problems', such as weakness, poor dexterity, discomfort – which can range from mild stiffness to severe, uncontrollable and very painful muscle spasms – and abnormal postures.[11]
- Damage to the part of the brain that processes information can cause 'cognitive impairment'. The survivor is less able to think clearly, remember things, solve problems and plan.[12] Survivors with cognitive problems may lose keys and shopping lists, miss

appointments or forget where they left a supermarket trolley or parked a car. We all do this from time to time. However, these problems can become worse after a stroke. Do not write the changes off as ageing or stress; rather, you ought to see your doctor. There are plenty of ways to give your mental abilities a boost (see page 70).

• Areas deep in your brain ensure that you breathe, that your heart beats and that your digest your last meal without thinking about it, even when you are asleep.

A stroke's effects also depend on the extent of the damage. You may not even realize that you have had a very mild stroke, although doctors can see tell-tale signs on a brain scan. Extensive damage, on the other hand, can be fatal, result in a vegetative state – where the survivor is awake but does not show any signs of awareness – or trigger locked-in syndrome – where the survivor is conscious and aware, but completely paralysed. Most people with locked-in syndrome can only control their eye movement. Fortunately, vegetative states and locked-in syndrome are relatively rare after a stroke.

More than a computer

Your brain weighs just 1.3–1.4 kg (3 pounds) but contains about 100 billion cells – about half the number of stars in the Milky Way (our galaxy). Each nerve cell (neurone) connects with many others, across 'gaps' called synapses, forming vast networks and 'pathways' that link areas of brain. If you cut a brain open, areas dense in neurones look grey – literally your grey matter.

Neurones release chemical messengers that cross the synapses and influence the activity of other neurones. The integrated action of millions of neurones allows us to think, move and live. Many drugs act by mimicking or blocking the action of these chemical messengers, called neurotransmitters.

Not surprisingly, the brain uses a lot of energy. Your brain accounts for about 2 per cent of your body weight, but uses about 20 per cent of the glucose (the sugar that fuels your body's activities) in your blood. Without a rich supply of glucose, other nutrients and oxygen, the brain cells die.

Writers often compare a brain to a computer. Yet this is an insult to your brain, which makes even the most powerful super-computer look like an especially simple slide rule. A computer cannot yet create the next *Mona Lisa*, write the next *Ulysses* or compose the next hit single (nor do I think it ever will), let alone the next Bach concerto. The Google Brain program used a million 'neurones' and a billion connections to learn to recognize cats on the internet. Google Brain's achievement is technologically remarkable. But it needed a cluster of 16,000 computers to view 10 million images[13] to match a single toddler's innate performance. And, of course, a toddler rapidly learns to recognize more than cats.

Unlike a computer, your brain is not hard-wired: your cells and nerve circuits continually adapt as you learn new tricks, skills and facts. For instance, during pregnancy, a mother's brain shrinks by around 4 per cent to meet the baby's demands for energy. Mothers recover the loss within about six months of giving birth.[14] This flexibility means that other parts of your brain can take over from damaged areas. Stroke rehabilitation forges new connections and trains other parts of your brain to compensate for the damaged area. As a result, the improvement after rehabilitation is greater than would have otherwise happened.

The brain's organization

Open a computer and you can see parts with defined roles: the central processor, transistors, diodes, capacitors and so on. A computer geek can work out what the circuit does. Look at a slice of brain under a microscope and even an experienced scientist cannot tell from this alone what the web of cells does. Biologists work out an area's function by what goes wrong when it is damaged.

For instance, during the nineteenth century, several doctors – most famously Pierre Paul Broca, professor of anatomy at the University of Paris – found that damage to a small part of the brain robbed the person of the power of speech, although the person could still think and count. Broca's area, usually on the left side of the brain, helps control speech and language. Strokes that damage Broca's area can cause speech problems, which are among the most frustrating and devastating complications of a stroke for survivors and carers.

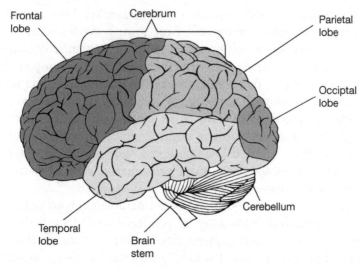

Figure 1.1 The main areas of the brain

By working backwards, by looking at autopsies of people with physical and mental problems, and by using a variety of other approaches, biologists gradually built up a map of the brain. A diagram of the main areas of the brain is shown in Figure 1.1. However, the brain is incredibly complex and the following are simplified examples. Anyone with a neurobiological background should probably look away.

The brainstem

The brainstem ensures that many basic biological functions – such as breathing, heart rate and swallowing – continue without us thinking about them, including while we are asleep. Other areas in the brainstem help with vision, hearing, balance, movement, the sleep–wake cycle, alertness and keeping our body at a constant temperature.

Strokes affecting the brainstem are, thankfully, rare.[15] Not surprisingly, strokes that damage a large part of the brainstem can prove fatal or leave the survivor in a vegetative state.[15] Even strokes that damage only a small part of the brainstem can cause debilitating problems with, for example, vision, balance and swallowing as well as weak or numb faces or limbs.[8]

When a stroke means that blue tastes disgusting

Some strokes cause remarkable changes. In *The Man Who Mistook His Wife for a Hat*, Oliver Sacks discusses an 'intelligent woman in her sixties' who after a massive stroke 'totally lost the idea of "left", both with regard to the world and her own body'. She put make up on the right half of her face, totally neglecting the left. She would complain that her meals were too small: she could not conceive that the plate had a left. She could not even turn left: she would move in a clockwise circle. Nurses and doctors could not draw her attention to the problem – she had no conception that anything was amiss. This is a dramatic example of a common problem (hemi-neglect) after a stroke: survivors cannot see or react to events on one side of their bodies. However, losing the entire concept of 'left' or 'right' is unusual.

In his fascinating book *Disturbances of the Mind*, Douwe Draaisma notes that strokes can trigger the enigmatic Capgras syndrome. Patients are convinced, often unshakeably, that an identical duplicate – a doppelganger, alien or robot – has replaced a loved one.

In another case, a Canadian stroke survivor developed synaesthesia – the 'merging' of senses. He experienced out-of-body experiences when listening to James Bond theme music and could taste colours. Apparently, blue tasted disgusting.

The cerebellum

The cerebellum (which literally means 'little brain') controls the timing and patterns of movement, helps you keep your balance as you move around, and aids co-ordination.[15,16] In particular, the cerebellum stores patterns of muscle movements. You call on the cerebellum when you take part in sport, for example, or play a musical instrument. Some studies suggest that playing certain instruments can aid stroke rehabilitation by helping people pay more attention to the damaged side of the body.[16] The cerebellum helps maintain posture by continually making fine adjustments to muscle tone. Not surprisingly, a stroke that damages the cerebellum can cause unsteadiness, poor co-ordination and clumsiness.[8]

The cerebrum

The cerebrum receives information from the rest of the body, including our senses. The cerebrum analyses the information, compares our current situation with our knowledge (including our experience, our formal education and what we have learnt in other ways) and decides if we need to take action. If we need to respond, the cerebrum sends messages to our muscles.[8]

The cerebrum consists of two 'halves' called hemispheres. Each hemisphere controls movement and other functions on the opposite side of the body. A stroke that damages areas of the right side of the brain affects movement on the left side of the body.

In most people, the right hemisphere also recognizes shapes, angles, proportions, patterns, faces and so on. The right side also controls emotions, creativity and imagination, and is responsible for your awareness of your body. The left hemisphere oversees analytical thought, problem solving, language, speech and understanding.

A thick cord of nerves connects the two hemispheres, which is one reason why the brain sometimes compensates for a stroke's effects: the area in the other hemisphere takes over. These dormant or underused regions 'light up' on a brain scan (see page 50) as they take over from areas damaged by the stroke.[7,8]

Each hemisphere has four lobes:[8,15]

- The occipital lobes control and process vision. A stroke affecting one of the occipital lobes can cause visual problems even though the eyes and the direct connections to the brain are healthy.
- The temporal lobes form and store long-term memories and are important for hearing and understanding speech.
- The parietal lobes confer our sense of space and perspective as well as receiving and interpreting information from our senses (such as touch and pressure) and contributing to speech.
- The frontal lobes influence personality, behaviour, decision-making, short-term memory and emotion, and are vital for movement and language.

The cardiovascular system

Your brain gets glucose, other nutrients and oxygen from a rich blood supply. Strokes arise from numerous causes – far more than result in a heart attack, for example. However, all the diverse causes interrupt the brain's blood supply.

The cardiovascular system refers to your blood vessels (arteries, veins and capillaries) and heart. Your brainstem ensures that, at rest, a healthy heart typically pumps 60 to 80 times a minute, 100,000 times every day,[17] or around three billion times in 80 years, rarely missing a beat.

Differences between arteries, veins and capillaries

Arteries carry blood away *from* the heart. Arteries branch into medium-sized and then small arteries (arterioles). In turn, arterioles divide into capillaries: a network of microscopic vessels inside all your body's tissues from your skin to your deepest internal organs. Capillaries' thin walls allow oxygen and nutrients to move from the blood into the cells. Meanwhile, blood in the capillaries absorbs carbon dioxide and other waste products. (In the lung, oxygen moves *into* the capillaries, while carbon dioxide moves out.) Capillaries merge, forming venules and, in turn, veins that return blood *to* the heart. Most arteries carry oxygen-rich blood. Most veins carry oxygen-depleted blood. However, pulmonary arteries carry oxygen-poor blood from your heart to your lungs. Pulmonary veins return oxygen-rich blood to your heart.

An average healthy heart – which is about the size of your fist and weighs approximately 0.3 kg (10 ounces) – pumps your 7 litres (12 pints) of blood along 96,500 kilometres (60,000 miles) of blood vessels.[17] Incredibly, if you laid your blood vessels end-to-end they would go around the equator almost two and a half times. Even at rest, a healthy heart pumps approximately 11,000 litres (2,500 gallons) of blood every day, shifting an Olympic swimming pool's worth of blood in about nine months.

The heart's four chambers – two atria and two ventricles (see Fig. 1.2 overleaf) – beat in sequence, pushing blood around two circulatory systems that begin and end at the heart (see Fig. 1.3 overleaf):

- the pulmonary circulation, which connects your heart to your lungs; and
- the systemic circulation, which connects your heart to all other parts of your body, including through the cerebral blood vessels to your head.

The atria collect blood from the pulmonary and systemic circulations. When they contract, the atria push blood into the ventricles. The two atria are smaller than the larger, stronger ventricles, with

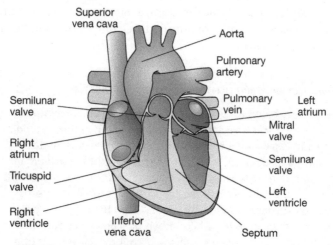

Figure 1.2   The structure of the heart

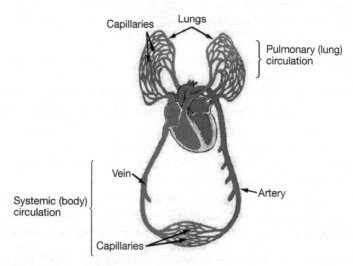

Figure 1.3   The circulatory system

thinner, less muscular walls. Nevertheless, atria help the ventricles work effectively. Some diseases affecting the atrias' performance – such as atrial fibrillation (see page 35) – mean that the heart does not pump blood properly. As we shall see, atrial fibrillation is an increasingly important cause of stroke.

The ventricles push blood around the thousands of miles of blood vessels. The right ventricle pumps blood to the lungs. The left ventricle pumps blood around the systemic circulation, including to the head through the cerebral circulation. So, the left ventricle is more muscular than the right ventricle. The septum divides the left and right sides of the heart. A 'hole in the heart' runs through the septum. One type of a hole of the heart – called a patent foramen ovale – is more common than many people realize, and can cause strokes (see page 22).

Heart valves ensure that blood flows in the correct direction (see Fig. 1.2):

- The tricuspid valve controls the flow between the right atrium and the right ventricle.
- The bicuspid (mitral) valve controls the flow between the left atrium and left ventricle.
- Semilunar valves, which remind biologists of a 'half moon', prevent blood pumped into the arteries from flowing back into the ventricles.

Occasionally, a clot (also called a thrombus) forms on these valves. Fragments of these clots can become lodged in the cerebral circulation, which potentially triggers a stroke (see page 22).

Inside your lungs

After entering your mouth and nose, air flows along your trachea, which is about 10–16 centimetres (four to six inches) long and around 2 centimetres (just less than an inch) wide. Horseshoe-shaped rings of cartilage – rather like the rings on a vacuum cleaner hose – protect the trachea from crushing. The trachea forks into two major bronchi, one supplying each lung. Each major bronchus divides another 10–25 times into bronchi and then bronchioles. The bronchioles end in between 300 million and 500 million alveoli, which look like cauliflower florets. This shape packs a vast area into a relatively small space. Overall, our lungs contain approximately 2,400 kilometres (1,500 miles) of airways. An adult's alveoli surface area is about 70 square metres – roughly the same as a single tennis court. A network of around 620 miles of capillaries surrounds the alveoli.

In the lungs, carbon dioxide moves from the blood into the alveoli. We expel toxic carbon dioxide when we breathe out. Meanwhile, oxygen in the air we have breathed in moves from the alveoli and attaches to an iron-rich protein (haemoglobin) in red blood cells. So, a diet that is low in iron can cause anaemia and exacerbate fatigue (see page 115), which is common after a stroke. Oxygen-rich blood travels from the lung through four pulmonary veins to the left atrium.

The muscular left ventricle pumps blood into the ascending aorta (see Fig. 1.2). From here, blood takes one of four routes:

- The coronary arteries – although the atria and ventricles are full of blood, a network of vessels supplies the heart muscle with oxygen and nutrients. Coronary heart disease (also called ischaemic heart disease) most commonly occurs when an accumulation of fat (see page 18) narrows these arteries. Most heart attacks occur after this accumulation triggers a clot that stops the blood flow and the area supplied by the vessel dies.
- The thoracic aorta, which supplies blood to organs in the chest, the head, the arms and hands.
- The abdominal aorta, which supplies blood to organs between the chest and pelvis as well as the legs and feet.
- Carotid arteries carry blood along the neck to the brain and into the cerebral blood vessels.

The cerebral circulation

The network of cerebral blood vessels is approximately 700 kilometres (about 430 miles) long – that's about the distance between Southampton and Glasgow. Most of these blood vessels are tiny capillaries,[18] although two systems of arteries supply the brain with blood:

- The carotid system. Once it reaches the middle of the neck, the common carotid artery splits. The internal carotid artery carries most of the blood to the brain. The external carotid artery supplies the face and scalp.[8]
- The vertebrobasilar system. Two vertebral arteries inside the backbone join at the base of the brain to form the basilar artery. This supplies blood to the cerebellum, the inner part and back of the cerebral hemispheres and other structures deep in the brain.[8]

More than plumbing

Your circulatory system is your body's largest organ: taken together, your blood vessels weigh about five times more than your heart. And your blood vessels are more than simple pipes. The walls of a blood vessel consist of three layers, which allow the vessel to respond to your body's demands:

- The tunica intima, the smooth inner lining that covers the inside of the blood vessel. Stripped off and laid flat, the tunica intima from throughout your body would cover a football pitch, while 350 layers stacked one of top of another could fit in the eye of a needle. Yet despite being microscopically thin, the tunica intima is remarkably resilient.
- The tunica media, the middle layer, which controls the vessel's diameter and maintains its flexibility.
- The tunica adventitia (also called tunica externa), which maintains the vessel's shape, limits distension and anchors the vessel.

Blood vessels tend to be narrower in the legs to maintain the pressure needed to get blood back to the heart. In contrast, the cerebral circulation is relatively dilated to slow down the flow and ensure the brain gets sufficient oxygen and nutrients.[19]

These vessels give rise to the three main cerebral arteries that supply the brain:

- the middle cerebral artery
- the posterior cerebral artery and
- the anterior cerebral artery.

Depending on the position and the severity of the blockage, a doctor may refer to, for example:

- a posterior stroke, a stroke in the area of the brain supplied by the posterior cerebral artery;
- a total anterior stroke, in which the anterior cerebral artery is completely blocked.

A total anterior stroke has a dreadful prognosis. More than half of people die within a year of developing this type of stroke. Almost all the survivors have marked disabilities.[3]

A lacunar stroke arises in one of the vessels supplying the deeper areas of the brain.[20] Blockages of these small vessels cause about a quarter of strokes. Because they affect a relatively small area of the brain, lacunar strokes can cause, for example, movement problems without affecting sensation, speech or vision. Age-related changes to medium and, especially, small arteries are one reason why strokes become more common as you get older.[3]

The carotid and vertebrobasilar systems join at the base of the brain forming the circle of Willis. This means that if an artery in the carotid or vertebrobasilar system becomes blocked, enough blood usually arrives through the circle of Willis to compensate. In addition, arteries in the brain can form branches that connect and bypass the blockage that caused the stroke. This collateral circulation helps restore the blood supply.[8] So, what goes wrong when someone experiences a stroke?

2

Causes and types of stroke

The term 'stroke' evokes a sudden, seemingly random blow: 'the stroke of God's hand' according to a sixteenth-century book.[21] Similarly, the older term for severe stroke – 'apoplexy' – derives from the Greek word for a 'violent blow'.[7] As the 1820 medical textbook *Treatise on Nervous Diseases* comments, a patient with apoplexy 'falls to the ground, often suddenly, and lies without sense or voluntary motion . . . as if struck by lightning'.[21] A stroke's sudden, violent appearance gives patients, the main carer – such as the husband, wife or partner – and other family members little time to prepare for an event that might turn their lives and relationships upside down. So, why does this often devastating disease strike hundreds of people each day?

Anita's story

Anita, a 58-year-old overweight grandmother, fell asleep in front of the television one Sunday afternoon. When she woke, Anita could not get up from the sofa: she kept falling back. When her husband helped her up, she noticed that she could not put any weight on her left foot. Anita said it was 'just a funny turn'. However, her husband noticed that the left side of her face seemed to droop, her speech was slightly slurred and she 'couldn't quite smile'. He called for an ambulance. An hour after she arrived in the accident and emergency department, her voice and face were normal, but she still felt weak. After a night in hospital, she was back to normal. The doctor told that she had suffered a TIA and needed to tackle her unhealthy lifestyle.

A common problem

Anita is not alone. Worldwide, about 15 million people suffer strokes every year. Almost six million die. Strokes leave another five million permanently disabled.[22] The elderly are most vulnerable: 83 per cent of deaths from stroke during 2010 in the UK occurred in people aged 75 years or older.

Potentially, however, almost anyone could suffer a stroke. Each year, about one in every 20,000 children in the UK has a stroke, while approximately 25 per cent of strokes occur in people under the age of 65 years.[20] However, some people are especially vulnerable:

- People from African Caribbean backgrounds are about twice as likely to have a stroke as white people and, on average, tend to have strokes at a younger age than white people. Doctors do not fully understand why black people are at increased risk. However, dangerously raised blood pressure (hypertension; see page 30), diabetes (see page 39) and sickle cell disease (see page 38) increase stroke risk and are more common in African Caribbean people than white people.

- People in the most deprived parts of the UK are around three times more likely to die prematurely from a stroke than those in the most affluent areas. Several factors link strokes and poverty, including a less healthy diet, higher levels of smoking and a more stressful life.

- Men are about 25 per cent more likely to suffer a stroke than women, according to the Stroke Association. However, women usually live longer. So, overall, more women suffer a stroke than men.

Types of stroke

Strokes can arise from a wide range of underlying problems, from the common to the extremely rare. However, there are, broadly, two main types:

About 85 per cent of strokes are ischaemic. In other words, an interruption or reduction in the blood supply (usually due to a clot) in an artery starves the brain of oxygen and nutrients. So, the brain cells supplied by that vessel die. Ischaemic strokes are less likely to be fatal than haemorrhagic strokes and many of the risk factors can be treated or managed.[15,20]

About 15 per cent strokes are 'intracerebral haemorrhages'. (Intracerebral means inside the head.) A blood vessel bursts and blood floods into, and destroys, part of the brain. Poorly managed or uncontrolled hypertension is the main risk factor for haemorrhagic strokes. Often, surgery to stop the bleeding, relieve the pressure and bypass the burst blood vessel is the only treatment.[15,20]

Table 2.1   Types of stroke

Stroke type	Stroke class	Per cent of strokes
Atherosclerosis of large arteries	Ischaemic	50
Lacunar strokes	Ischaemic	25
Blood clot forms in the heart and travels to the brain (embolism)	Ischaemic	20
Primary intracerebral haemorrhage	Haemorrhagic	10
Subarachnoid haemorrhage	Haemorrhagic	5
Rare causes (e.g. arterial dissection, patent foramen ovale)	Ischaemic	5

Adapted from the Stroke Association

About 12 per cent of strokes are cryptogenic.[20] Doctors use this term when they do not know what caused the stroke.

Strokes in children and younger adults often arise from different causes – such as abnormalities in arteries, infections, cancers and meningitis – from those in the typical stroke patient.[7] However, according to the Stroke Association, doctors cannot identify a cause for stroke in a third of younger adults.

Doctors subdivide ischaemic and haemorrhagic strokes (see Table 2.1). You may not recognize the names, although you will by the end of the chapter.

Transient ischaemic attacks (TIAs) – heed the mini-stroke warning

Each year, one person in every 1000 has a TIA,[3] where a short-lived blood clot interrupts the blood flow to part of the brain or the eye. This starves the brain or the light-sensitive layer at the back of the eye (the retina) of blood. When the TIA affects the blood supply to the retina, the person can experience blindness in one eye that lasts for several seconds to a few minutes.[5,7,15] When the TIA affects the blood supply to the brain, the patient can develop typical signs of a stroke, such as weakness, slurred speech and facial droop.

Nevertheless, TIAs can prove difficult to diagnose. About half of people referred to a specialist with a suspected TIA turn out to have another condition, such as migraine (see page 45), a brain tumour or multiple sclerosis.[3]

Following a TIA, the body restores the blood supply relatively rapidly. As a result, TIA symptoms often last only a few minutes, resolve totally within 24 hours and do not produce long-lasting physical, cognitive or mental problems.[23] For example, symptoms lasted less than 10 minutes in almost a quarter of TIA patients interviewed by the Stroke Association. However, the survey showed that about 70 per cent of people reported long-term effects after the TIA, including memory loss (experienced by 41% of those interviewed), muscle weakness (38%), confusion (26%), poor mobility (25%), and problems with speech (21%) and understanding (18%). But a fine line divides a TIA from a mild stroke. Many persistent changes produced by a mild stroke are subtle and doctors treat TIAs in essentially the same way.[3]

A TIA or mild stroke is usually a warning that you have atherosclerosis (see page 18) in the blood vessels supplying your brain. Occasionally, however, an embolism (see page 22) or a small haemorrhage causes symptoms that are indistinguishable from a TIA.[5] Over time, this atherosclerosis can get worse and, eventually, you could suffer a devastating stroke that produces lasting disability or even proves fatal.

Indeed, around one person in 50 who experiences a TIA has a stroke within the next two days. One in 20 has a stroke within seven days. Overall, about a quarter of people who have an ischaemic stroke have a TIA first.[3] Your risk of a stroke is especially high if you:

- experience crescendo TIA – more than two episodes in a week;[5]
- have atrial fibrillation (see page 35); or
- are taking anticoagulants (see page 52).[5]

On the other hand, the Stroke Association notes that treating TIA urgently reduces the risk of a stroke by 80 per cent. This underscores, once again, why you must get medical help as soon as you develop any symptoms that might indicate a stroke.

Get the help you need

Despite the importance of rapid treatment, many people who experience TIA symptoms put off getting the help they need. The Stroke Association interviewed 670 people who experienced a TIA. The report *Not just a funny turn* makes disturbing reading:

- 20 per cent of people who experienced a TIA went on to suffer a major stroke;
- 47 per cent said that the TIA's symptoms 'didn't feel like an emergency';
- 37 per cent thought that the mini-stroke was a 'funny turn';
- Only 22 per cent of those experiencing symptoms rang 999;
- 14 per cent took no action;
- About 10 per cent said that they delayed taking action because they did not know whom to contact.

In other words, never ignore symptoms that could indicate a stroke or TIA. Do not dismiss the symptoms as fatigue, a trapped nerve, migraine or just a funny turn. If in doubt, call 999 or ask someone to drive you to the accident and emergency department as soon as possible.

A condition surrounded by ignorance

Despite several high-profile campaigns, the report *Not just a funny turn* shows that many people do not appreciate a TIA's significance. Before experiencing a mini-stroke, 44 per cent of those interviewed by the Stroke Association had never heard of TIA. Another 27 per cent had heard of TIA, but did not know a lot about the condition. Furthermore, 61 per cent were unaware that a TIA is a warning of a possible future stroke.

Given this widespread ignorance, in case you experience a TIA you should make sure that everyone – family, friends and colleagues – knows what to watch for and appreciates the importance of calling 999 immediately if you show symptoms of a stroke or TIA. If you are a manager, you could consider educating your staff about TIAs and strokes. After all, strokes and TIAs can strike almost anyone out of the blue.

If you suffer a TIA, you need to discuss the best way to reduce your risk of stroke, heart attacks and other cardiovascular diseases with your doctor. A healthy lifestyle and drugs to, for example, control hypertension and prevent clots, should help reduce your risk of a full-blown stroke.[23] However, as mentioned in the introduction, almost a quarter of people who experience a TIA said that health-care professionals did not give them advice about the important lifestyle changes. So, you might need to ask – but don't wait.

Two groups of stroke symptoms

Doctors and nurses divide symptoms into two broad groups:

- Focal symptoms arise from damage to a specific, identifiable area of the brain. Weakness or altered sensations on one side of the body and speech disorders are focal symptoms. Strokes cause most – but not all – focal symptoms seen by healthcare professionals.[20]
- Non-focal symptoms – such as dizziness or generalized weakness – cannot be traced to a specific area of the brain. Many diseases other than stroke can cause non-focal symptoms. Indeed, stroke is a relatively uncommon cause of non-focal symptoms.[20]

The characteristic focal symptoms arise because the stroke stops parts of the brain from working properly. This usually causes 'negative symptoms' such as weakness or loss of vision, balance or feeling. 'Positive symptoms', such as flashing lights or pins and needles, generally arise from other problems, such as migraine or a trapped nerve.[7] However, you should call 999 if you experience any symptom on page ix.

Ischaemic strokes

Around 500 years ago, Leonardo da Vinci noticed that a layer of 'waxy fat' covered blood vessels supplying elderly people's hearts. Today, we know that fat starts collecting *inside* arteries from early childhood – perhaps even while we are in the womb. This accumulation – called atherosclerosis – in a large blood vessel causes about half of ischaemic strokes.[7]

'Sclerosis' means hardening, and *athere* is the Greek word for 'gruel' or 'porridge', which gives you an idea of the consistency. I'll never forget the film at a medical conference where a heart surgeon ran his finger along the outside of an artery with severe atherosclerosis. Fat ran out of the end as if he was squeezing toothpaste from a tube.

A plaque's development

Most plaques – the name doctors give to an atherosclerotic deposit – start developing at around 25 years of age and usually take between 10 and 15 years to mature fully. As a plaque enlarges, the lumen

(a) Healthy artery

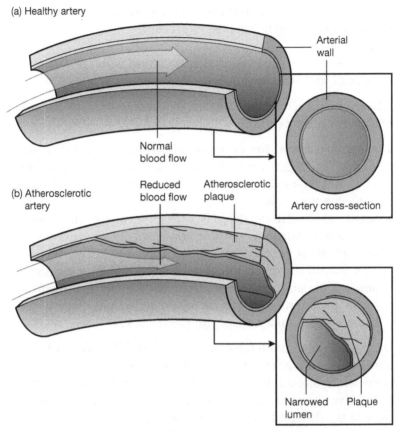

Figure 2.1   Atherosclerotic plaques can narrow the lumen of an artery

(the size of the 'bore' down the middle of the vessel) narrows (see Fig. 2.1). This reduces blood flow, which can cause a range of health problems depending on the site of the plaque.

Atherosclerosis begins as smears of fat that form around damage to the tunica intima – the blood vessel's normally smooth inner lining (see page 11). Numerous factors can sow the seeds of atherosclerosis, including:

- particularly turbulent blood flow – for instance, blood flow is turbulent where medium and large blood vessels branch, such as where the common carotid splits into the internal and external branches (see page 10);[8]

- excessive levels of fat in the blood (dyslipidaemia);
- raised sugar levels in the blood (diabetes);
- hypertension;
- changes to the blood vessels that are linked with age;
- nicotine and other toxins from smoking.

Atherosclerosis can emerge almost anywhere in the cardiovascular system. For instance:

- Atherosclerosis in the major vessels supplying the brain cause strokes. The bigger the vessel, the greater the area of brain supplied and, as a rule, the greater the risk of death and disability following the stroke.
- Small atherosclerotic deposits can form where small vessels branch from larger ones. These vessels supply a relatively small area. However, if this brain region happens to include a critical area, a small stroke can still be devastating. For example, a small amount of damage to nerves that send signals to the muscles in the face, arm or leg can cause severe paralysis. Nevertheless, death is less common than with larger strokes.[7]

Damage to the tunica intima allows fats and certain types of white blood cell (which normally fight infections) to enter the vessel wall. Some white blood cells become engorged with fat, forming foam cells. Meanwhile, chemical messengers released by white blood cells inflame the damaged area and increase the amount of muscle and collagen in the blood vessel wall. (Collagen, which accounts for a quarter of the protein in your body, enhances tissues' strength and flexibility.) The messengers recruit more white blood cells into the damaged area.

These changes 'patch' the damaged vessel wall. But it's a short-term 'fix'. Fat continues to pour from the blood into the plaque. Muscle cells form a cap covering a core of foam cells, lipid and debris from dead cells. Capillaries grow into the developing plaque. These newly formed vessels are fragile and blood leaks into, and further swells, the plaque. Calcium also accumulates in, and gradually hardens, the plaque.

At first, arteries enlarge to accommodate the plaque. But after the plaque occupies more than 40 per cent of the vessel wall, it begins to narrow the lumen and cuts blood flow. The plaques can burst,

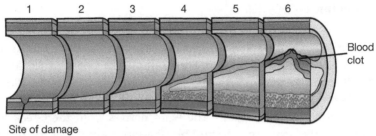

Site of damage

1 Damage to the inner lining of the blood vessel
2 Fatty streak forms at site of damage
3 Foam cells numbers increase, area is inflamed and small pools of fat appear
4 Large core of fat develops, and amounts of muscle and collagen increase
5 Fibrous cap covers a fat-rich core, while calcium deposits harden the plaque
6 Plaque ruptures triggering a blood clot

Figure 2.2   Development of an atherosclerotic plaque

spilling their contents into the blood. This triggers a blood clot that
may block the vessel and cause an ischaemic stroke or TIA (see Fig.
2.2). The process is the same as that causing most heart attacks,
and you will sometimes see strokes or TIAs called 'brain attacks'.[7]
In TIAs, the body manages to dissolve the clot before enough brain
cells die to cause irreversible problems.

Zones of damage

An ischaemic stroke produces two 'zones' of damage:

- In the 'core' zone, blood flow falls to less than 10–25 per cent of
  normal. The loss of oxygen and glucose rapidly kills brain cells.
- The penumbra refers to the area between the regions of the brain
  that receive a normal blood supply and the core zone. Cells in
  the penumbra receive blood from vessels surrounding the core
  zone.[24] The penumbra survives for a few minutes to several hours
  depending on the extent of this blood supply.[7] However, cells in
  the penumbra eventually die if the blood supply does not return
  to normal.[24]

A treatment called thrombolysis (see page 51) reduces the size of the
ischaemic penumbra by rapidly restoring the blood supply.[20] In other
words, seeking medical help as soon as you suspect something is
wrong can help reduce the amount of damage to your brain.

Embolism

In 20–35 per cent of ischaemic strokes, a fragment of a blood clot (thromboembolism) that formed elsewhere in the body blocks an artery supplying the brain.[25] For example, in people with atrial fibrillation (see page 35) the heart does not pump properly. Blood left behind in the heart can clot. Fragments of this clot can break off, forming an embolism – the word derives from the Greek for 'throw' – that can travel to and block arteries supplying the brain, causing a stroke. Similarly, emboli in an artery supplying the kidney can cause part of this essential organ to die. Emboli in a major vessel supplying the legs can cause gangrene.[7]

Embolisms can also arise from a deep vein thrombosis (DVT), which occurs when a blood clot forms in a vein in the lower leg, thigh, pelvis or, less commonly, the arm.[26] A part of the clot can break off and reaches the blood vessels supplying the brain, causing an ischaemic stroke.

More commonly, the fragment travels to the lungs, causing a blockage called a pulmonary embolism. A large pulmonary embolism can stop the supply of blood to the lung, which can prove fatal. Indeed, pulmonary embolisms kill about 15 per cent of people with an untreated DVT and are an 'important cause of early death after stroke'.[26] We shall look at some ways of preventing DVTs and pulmonary emboli in Chapter 4.

A hole in the heart

Normally, vessels in the lung filter small clots from the circulation before blood reaches the arteries supplying the brain. However, around a quarter of people have a type of hole in the heart (called a patent foramen ovale) caused when the septum (see page 9) does not close properly after birth.[5]

A developing baby gets oxygen and nutrients from its mother across the placenta. The foramen ovale allows blood to bypass the lungs while the baby is developing in the womb. The foramen ovale usually closes completely in the year after birth.[7] However, in people with patent foramen ovale, the hole allows blood to bypass the lung filter, which makes a stroke caused by an embolism more likely.

Hereditary haemorrhagic telangiectasia

A rare condition called hereditary haemorrhagic telangiectasia causes enlarged blood vessels in the lungs. This enlargement, which is similar to varicose veins, means that the vessels do not filter clots from the blood as efficiently as in healthy people, which increases the likelihood of suffering a stroke.

Haemorrhagic strokes

During a haemorrhagic stroke, a blood vessel supplying the brain bursts. Blood floods into the brain. These 'primary intra-cerebral haemorrhages' cause about 13 per cent of strokes overall, but between 40 and 50 per cent in younger adults, the Stroke Association notes. However, the amount of blood released during a haemorrhagic stroke varies widely. A micro-bleed (see page 24) usually does not cause symptoms, whereas a large haemorrhagic stroke can rapidly kill.[7] As a rule, however, haemorrhagic strokes are more severe and cause more deaths than ischaemic strokes.[3]

Haemorrhagic strokes have three main causes:[7]

• weakened or damaged blood vessels – such as an aneurysm (see page 25);
• blood that does not clot properly;
• blood pressure that is too high (hypertension), which can weaken or damage blood vessels.[7]

Subarachnoid haemorrhage

Vessels in or near the membranes (the meninges) that cover the brain and spinal cord can burst, causing a type of stroke called a subarachnoid haemorrhage. The meninges consist of three layers:

• the pia mater, which is the membrane closest to the brain or spinal cord;
• the dura mater, which is on the outside, just under the skull or next to the bones in the spine; and
• the arachnoid layer, which is sandwiched between the pia mater and the dura mater.

During a subarachnoid haemorrhage, a burst vessel bleeds into the space beneath the arachnoid layer.[20]

The symptoms of a subarachnoid haemorrhage may differ from ischaemic and primary intracerebral haemorrhagic strokes.[3] You should phone 999 if you experience one or more of the following:

- a sudden agonizing headache – many people describe the pain as like being suddenly hit on the head, and say that the blinding pain is unlike anything they have experienced before;
- a stiff neck;
- nausea and vomiting that you cannot explain;
- over-sensitivity to light;
- blurred or double vision;
- confusion;
- other stroke symptoms, such as slurred speech and weakness on one side of the body;
- unconsciousness;
- convulsions (uncontrollable shaking).

Subarachnoid haemorrhages account for about 6 per cent of strokes overall,[20] but about 80 per cent occur in women. The outlook is often poor. However, the sooner you get help the better your chances.

- 10–15 per cent of people with subarachnoid haemorrhages die before they reach hospital;
- around 25 per cent die within 24 hours of the subarachnoid haemorrhage;
- overall, only about half survive;
- half the survivors will have disability and most will experience chronic (long-lasting) symptoms, such as fatigue and cognitive problems.[5]

Micro-bleeds

Sometimes vessels burst, but only a small amount of blood enters the brain or the subarachnoid space. These 'micro-bleeds' seem to be relatively common, occurring in, for example, 10–20 per cent of elderly people. Micro-bleeds do too little damage to cause symptoms – doctors identify them only on a brain scan for another reason. However, people who have micro-bleeds are more likely to go on to have a full-blown haemorrhagic stroke.[27] For example, about a third of people who have a subarachnoid haemorrhage had a minor bleed before it.[8]

Aneurysm

An aneurysm is a 'pouch' or 'ballooning' of an artery, usually where the blood vessel's lining is weaker. About 95 per cent of cerebral (in the head) aneurysms do not cause symptoms. However, the weakness means that the aneurysm can burst, often when blood pressure reaches a short-lived peak, such as during strong emotions, heavy lifting, coughing, sex and even urination and defaecation.[5,28] Aneurysms can also form elsewhere in the body. For example, weak heart muscle can form a 'pocket' called a ventricular aneurysm. Clots are more likely to form in these pockets and fragments can travel to the vessels supplying the brain.

Overall, about 85 per cent of subarachnoid haemorrhages occur when a cerebral aneurysm bursts.[5] The initial bleed from an aneurysm may last only seconds. However, further bleeding is common and, if persistent, can lead to coma and death.[28] Tragically, around 10 per cent of patients who experience a ruptured aneurysm die before reaching hospital. Forty per cent of those who reach hospital will die within the next 30 days. A third of survivors show persistent disability.[28]

The risk of rupture

So, how likely are aneurysms to rupture? To answer this, researchers followed 118 people with intracranial aneurysms that had not yet ruptured. They followed each person for the rest of his or her life or until the person had a subarachnoid haemorrhage. On average, doctors diagnosed the aneurysm when the person was about 44 years old. Twenty-nine per cent of these people developed a subarachnoid haemorrhage, which occurred, on average, at around 51 years of age.[29]

On average, one in every 63 aneurysms burst each year. However, aneurysms of at least 7 mm (about a quarter of an inch) were about 14 times more likely to rupture in women and almost twice as likely to burst in men than smaller ones. Nevertheless, quarter of people with aneurysms of less than 7 mm experienced a subarachnoid haemorrhage.[29]

Overall, aneurysms (of any size) were 2.5 times more likely to burst in women than men. Doctors do not fully understand why aneurysms are more likely to occur and to burst in women than men. Smoking increased the risk of subarachnoid haemorrhages by almost 3.5 times. Systolic blood pressure over 140 mmHg doubled the risk.[29] We shall look at ways to quit smoking and reduce blood pressure later.

Systolic and diastolic blood pressure

Systole refers to the contraction of the heart's chambers. Diastole is the relaxation between beats, when the chambers fill with blood. So, doctors and nurses record systolic and diastolic blood pressure. The top number is the peak systolic blood pressure, the bottom the lowest diastolic pressure. So, if you have a blood pressure of 140/95, 140 mmHg is the systolic pressure and 95 mmHg the diastolic.

Surgery can strengthen an aneurysm, although sometimes the risks outweigh the benefits.[8] However, if you have two or more close relatives (parent, sibling or child) who have an aneurysm or if you have polycystic renal disease you are at increased risk of having an aneurysm.[5] You should talk to your GP to see if it is worth being screened and, if you have an aneurysm, discuss the risks and benefits of surgery with a specialist.

Arteriovenous malformation

An arteriovenous malformation (AVM) is a tangled network of high-pressure arteries linked directly to low-pressure veins. The AVM lacks the usual intervening network of capillaries that dissipates the pressure. This places the AVM under considerable strain.

About one in 1000 people have an AVM,[28] which can occur anywhere in the body. AVMs probably arise when the circulatory system does not develop normally in the womb or soon after birth. As the person gets older, the AVM grows, becomes weaker and more prone to bleeding. As a result, an AVM in the brain can cause epilepsy, haemorrhage, stroke, severe disability or death. Bleeding from an AVM tends to be less abrupt than with an aneurysm, but the haemorrhage can persist for longer.[28]

AVMs and other abnormalities in blood vessels cause around 5 per cent of subarachnoid haemorrhages.[5] On average, one in 50 AVMs bleeds for the first time each year. Eventually, about half of AVMs bleed. One in five AVMs bursts again in the following year. Between 3.5 and 9.3 per cent of AVMs rupture during pregnancy.

In other words, the risk is higher than when you're not pregnant. The risk seems to peak during the second trimester.[28] In addition, about 60 per cent of people with an AVM have an aneurysm within it or near to it.[28]

Life after a stroke

As mentioned above, once you survive a stroke, you are vulnerable to having another. For example, when researchers combined 13 studies that included 9115 patients, they found that:[4]

- about 3 per cent of people who survived their first stroke experience a recurrence within 30 days;
- within a year, 11 per cent have another stroke;
- within five years of their first stroke, around 26 per cent have another stroke;
- within ten years of their first stroke, about 39 per cent have another stroke.

In addition, strokes cause more disabilities and a greater range of disabilities than any other chronic (long-term) disease. As Table 2.2 indicates, fewer than half of survivors are independent and almost a quarter have severe or very severe disabilities. Nevertheless, many people regain a considerable amount of their function and can adapt their lifestyle and surroundings to compensate. Just because you have survived a stroke, does not mean you will not be able to live a full and active life.

Table 2.2   Level of disability among stroke survivors

Level of disability	Per cent of survivors affected
Independent	42
Mild	22
Moderate	14
Severe	10
Very severe	12

Adapted from the Stroke Association

Young people and strokes

As we have seen (see page 15), the causes of stroke in children and young adults often differ from those in older people. Furthermore, young adults tend to have different rehabilitation needs partly because they face specific issues, such as a greater economic need to get back to work or having to bring up children. In addition, problems with families or relationships can have a greater impact. And older people can often draw on lessons they have learned during other difficult experiences to help them cope.

Tragically, strokes leave many young people facing marked disability. Researchers looked at 722 people who experienced their first stroke between 18 and 50 years. On average nine years after the stroke, about one-third needed help for some activities, such as caring for themselves, doing household chores or looking after finances.[30]

The 91 patients in this study who experienced another stroke fared especially badly: 55 per cent of those who suffered at least one more stroke needed help with some activities, compared with 29 per cent of those who did not experience another stroke. Furthermore, 33 per cent of those who had more than one stroke depended on others for the activities of daily living, compared with 12 per cent of those without a second stroke.[30] This underscores the importance of taking steps to prevent another stroke, whatever your age.

3

Risk factors for stroke

Flick through any medical textbook and you will see a daunting list of risk factors for stroke. After all, 'stroke' is an umbrella term encompassing a variety of causes from the very widespread to the extremely rare. We cannot cover every risk factor. But this chapter looks at the most common.

The 'classic' stroke risk factors – such as increasing age, hypertension, smoking, diabetes and heart disease – cause 50 to 60 per cent of strokes.[31] In addition, lack of physical activity, obesity, high cholesterol, poor diet, stress and depression, and high alcohol intake all increase the likelihood of a stroke. You can't modify your age, of course. However, you can take steps to modify the other ten factors, which together account for almost 90 per cent of the risk of having a stroke.[15]

What is a risk factor?

A risk factor increases your chance of developing a particular disease. For example, smoking is a risk factor for many cancers, obesity is a risk factor for knee osteoarthritis, and drinking too much alcohol is a risk factor for liver disease. However, having one or more risk factors does not mean that the disease is inevitable – everyone seems to have a relative who smoked, ate an unhealthy diet and drank heavily and yet died at a ripe old age.

You may also develop the disease without having a common risk factor: according to Cancer Research UK, 14 per cent of lung cancers are not caused by active or passive smoking. Most cardiovascular events – such as strokes and heart attacks – occur in people who doctors do *not* regard as being at high risk.[3] That's why a healthy lifestyle is important for everyone: you may still reduce your likelihood of a disease even your doctor doesn't tell you you're at high risk.

The factors are cumulative: your risk worsens if, for example, you are hypertensive and smoke, and worsens again if you are hypertensive, smoke and have diabetes. On the other hand, few people have no modifiable risk factors. So, even if you have a risk factor you cannot change (such as getting older or your ethnic background) tackling those you can do something about reduces your overall likelihood of suffering a stroke and helps prevent recurrence.

Hypertension (dangerously high blood pressure)

As mentioned in Chapter 1, your heart pushes blood along thousands of miles of vessels. Not surprisingly, this takes considerable force. Indeed, across the animal kingdom, blood pressure varies depending on the distance blood has to travel, from just 15 mmHg in some worms to a systolic pressure of 260 mmHg in a giraffe.[19] The latter's high pressure gets enough blood to the brain to prevent the Serengeti from becoming home to towers of fainting giraffes.

Blood pressure is a measure of the force exerted against the artery walls. In turn, blood pressure depends on the force generated by the heart, the amount of blood pumped around the circulation, and the size and flexibility of the arteries. Arteries become stiffer as we get older. This and other age-related changes in blood vessels are one reason why stroke becomes more common as we age.

You need sufficient blood pressure to ensure that all your tissues receive the oxygen and nutrients they need. As a result, blood pressure is higher when you walk around than when you lounge on the sofa. Blood pressure increases again when you run for the bus or chase after the kids in the park.

In some people, however, blood pressure remains excessively high for too long, which increases the risk of strokes, other cardiovascular diseases and dementia.[27] Their blood pressure remains elevated when they are just sitting or lying down rather than exercising – in other words, they have hypertension.

Hypertension rarely causes symptoms – although if you suffer any of the symptoms in Table 3.1 you should see a doctor urgently. These could be a sign of an especially dangerous form of raised blood pressure called malignant hypertension. Some of these symptoms overlap with those of stroke, which is another good reason to get them checked.

Table 3.1   Symptoms that could indicate malignant hypertension

Confusion

Changes in vision

Fatigue

Headache – especially if severe

Irregular heartbeat

Nosebleed, without injury

Tinnitus (unexplained buzzing or noise in the ears)

Measuring blood pressure

Doctors and nurses measure blood pressure in millimetres of mercury (mmHg) using a sphygmomanometer, introduced by the Italian doctor Scipione Riva-Rocci in 1896. Physicists originally measured the pressure exerted by fluids by seeing how far a column of mercury moved. The technique for measuring blood pressure has changed. However, the unit of measurement remains the same.

Until recently, doctors and nurses used a stethoscope to listen for the 'Korotkoff' sounds made by the changing blood flow in the artery as the cuff deflates. Today, most doctors and nurses use automatic sphygmomanometers to measure the peak systolic pressure and lowest diastolic pressure (see page 26). Increasingly, however, doctors diagnose hypertension following 24-hour ambulatory blood pressure monitoring (ABPM) rather than on the basis of a couple of readings in the surgery. You wear a device that continually measures your blood pressure over the day. ABPM diagnoses hypertension more accurately and reduces unnecessary treatments.

The hazards of hypertension

According to the Stroke Association, hypertension contributes to about half of all strokes. Over time, hypertension changes blood vessels' structure so they are better able to resist the increased pressure. For example, the vessels' walls become thicker, stronger and stiffer. While this reduces the risk of damage, the changes tend to maintain high blood pressure.[27]

After a point, the thicker, stronger and stiffer vessels become more brittle. So, the vessel is less able to cope with a sudden increase in blood pressure from exercise or emotion. (Healthy vessels are flexible enough to cope with the additional pressure.) These brittle vessels can burst, causing a haemorrhagic stroke. Hypertension can also damage the arteries' smooth inner lining, sowing the seed for atherosclerosis (see page 18), or it can trigger a plaque to burst, resulting in an ischaemic stroke.

The dangers of pre-hypertension

There is no clear point above which blood pressure suddenly becomes dangerous.[7] Indeed, increases in blood pressure that are only just above normal – so-called pre-hypertension – seem to increase stroke risk by 66 per cent compared with optimal blood pressure (less than 120/80 mmHg).[32] For example, after allowing for other cardiovascular risk factors, low-range pre-hypertension (120–129/80–84 mmHg) increases stroke risk by 44 per cent. High-range pre-hypertension (130–139/85–89 mmHg) increases stroke risk by 95 per cent.[32]

Although pre-hypertension might contribute to up to a fifth of strokes,[32] doctors do not always treat blood pressures at these levels. So, if you have had a stroke or are at increased risk, you might want to discuss treating pre-hypertension with your doctor, especially if lifestyle changes do not adequately reduce your blood pressure.

The mystery of hypertension

During 2012, according to the Health Survey for England, 31 per cent of men and 27 per cent of women either had hypertension or took drugs to lower blood pressure. But just 9% of both sexes had controlled hypertension. Furthermore, 16% of men and 11% of women had untreated hypertension.

Why so many people have hypertension and why raised blood pressure is so difficult to treat remain something of a mystery. Doctors can identify an underlying cause in only 5–10 per cent of cases, which they call secondary hypertension.[33] Numerous conditions can cause secondary hypertension, including:

- some kidney diseases;
- sleep apnoea (interruptions to breathing during sleep);
- white coat hypertension (see page 33);
- drinking excessive amounts of alcohol (see page 41);

- eating too much, or being abnormally sensitive to, salt (see page 88);
- being overweight (see page 109).

Treating secondary hypertension often lowers blood pressure to safe levels. Unfortunately, few people with hypertension have identifiable, treatable causes of their raised blood pressure.

White coat and white skirt hypertension

Some people seem to have hypertension when a doctor or nurse measures their blood pressure. Outside the clinic, however, anti-hypertensive medicines effectively control their hypertension or their blood pressure is normal without treatment. These people have 'white coat hypertension'. The 'stress' of the measurement drives blood pressure up. About 40 per cent of people taking one or two antihypertensives and almost 30 per cent of those on three show white coat hypertension.[34]

Furthermore, Japanese researchers found that when women measured the blood pressure of men aged 18–20 years, diastolic and systolic readings were, on average, 5 mmHg higher than when men made the recording. Almost 11 per cent of young men showed readings sufficient to diagnose hypertension when a woman measured blood pressure compared with 4 per cent when a man took the reading. The sex of the person measuring did not influence blood pressure or heart rate in females of the same age. The researchers called the phenomenon 'white skirt hypertension'.[35]

It might seem like a joke from *Carry on Doctor*, but white skirt hypertension eloquently illustrates the environment's effect on blood pressure. More seriously, some people with white coat hypertension may be taking antihypertensives that don't do them any good but that put them at risk of side-effects.[34] White coat hypertension is one reason why increasing numbers of doctors use ABPM before diagnosing hypertension.

As we shall see in Chapter 5, drugs (antihypertensives) and lifestyle changes can reduce blood pressure. However, antihypertensives are added to – and not a replacement for – lifestyle changes. Furthermore, a doctor or nurse should measure your blood pressure at least once a year. You can buy blood pressure monitors to use at home. However, seek advice first. For example, you need to make sure the monitor is accurate and you have the right-sized cuff. Your

GP or hospital, the British Heart Foundation or the Blood Pressure Association may be able to help you choose the best machine for you.

Lethal and healthy cholesterol

Despite its bad press, cholesterol is essential for health and well-being. Cholesterol, a type of fat, is a building block of the membranes that surround every cell. Cholesterol forms part of the insulation (myelin sheath) around many nerve fibres. This sheath ensures that nerve signals travel properly. Cholesterol is also the backbone of several hormones, including oestrogen, testosterone and progesterone. Unfortunately, poor diets and a lack of exercise (which burns fat) mean that many of us have too much of a good thing.

Transporting cholesterol and other fats around the body poses a biological conundrum. Blood is about four-fifths water. Oil (a type of fat that is liquid at room temperature) and water do not mix. So, your body surrounds the core of cholesterol with a water-soluble coat made up of special chemicals called 'lipoproteins'. For example:

- Low-density lipoprotein (LDL) carries cholesterol from the liver to the tissues. LDL accumulates in artery walls, which contributes to atherosclerosis.
- High-density lipoprotein (HDL) carries between a quarter and a third of the cholesterol in the blood. HDL tends to carry cholesterol away from the arteries and back to the liver for excretion from the body. So, for example, HDL removes cholesterol from plaques in the walls of arteries, which slows atherosclerosis.

In other words, high levels of LDL increase the risk of heart attacks and strokes. High levels of HDL protect against cardiovascular disease. It's easy to remember: LDL is 'lethal'; HDL is 'healthy'.

Fat is also a concentrated source of energy – one gram of fat in the diet provides nine calories. A high-fat diet can contribute to people being overweight or obese, which increases the risk of diabetes, certain cancers, coronary heart disease and ischaemic strokes. Dietary changes (see page 94) and drugs (see page 58) can help reduce dangerous levels of cholesterol in your blood and keep your weight in check.

Arrhythmias

Usually the heart beats regularly and steadily, the pace changing to keep up with the demands we face. Sometimes, however, the heart-beat becomes irregular – a so-called arrhythmia.

Most arrhythmias are harmless, but some are serious or even life-threatening. For example, about 800,000 people in the UK have a type of arrhythmia doctors call atrial fibrillation. Another 250,000 people do not know they have the arrhythmia. In atrial fibrillation, the atria (see page 7) beat irregularly, usually, rapidly – sometimes contracting up to 400 times a minute – and quiver (fibrillate). Atrial fibrillation increases the risk of stroke up to five-fold and tends to trigger more severe strokes than many other risk factors.[3]

Atrial fibrillation becomes more common as we get older: about 7 per cent of people aged 65 years or over and 12 per cent of those aged 75 years or over have the arrhythmia. The growing number of elderly people means that atrial fibrillation is an increasingly common cause of stroke.[3]

So, why is atrial fibrillation dangerous? The rapid, irregular heart-beats give time for the chambers to only partly contract, and the actions of the atria and ventricles are uncoordinated. As a result, the amount of blood pumped by the heart falls by 15–20 per cent.[36] Because the heart pumps less effectively, people with atrial fibrillation may experience breathlessness (often the first symptom), palpitations and dizziness. Initially, a person typically experiences isolated attacks. Over time, however, atrial fibrillation usually becomes increasingly persistent.[37]

The poorly co-ordinated contractions mean that atrial fibrillation leaves some blood in the heart, where it can clot. The clots are especially likely to form in the left atrium. Fragments from these clots (embolisms) can travel in the circulation and block the blood vessels supplying the brain. Indeed, atrial fibrillation may underlie up to a quarter of strokes.[7,37]

According to NICE, patients with atrial fibrillation should receive anticoagulation (see page 52), which prevents blood clots. However, only 36 per cent of patients with known atrial fibrillation admitted to hospital with a stroke were taking anticoagulants. As we've seen (see page ix), NICE estimate that effective detection and protection with anticoagulant drugs could prevent around 7,000 strokes and 2,000 premature deaths.

So, ask your doctor or nurse to take your pulse. Everyone who has an irregular pulse should have an ECG whether or not they experience symptoms. You should also have your pulse taken if you experience breathlessness, palpitations or dizziness.

Clots on heart valves

As mentioned in Chapter 1, heart valves ensure that blood flows correctly through the heart. However, clots can form if the heart valves are:

- misshapen – for example, because of developmental problems in the womb;
- scarred – for example, from rheumatic heart disease; or
- artificial (after valve-replacement surgery).

For instance, about 6 per cent of people show 'mitral valve prolapse', in which the bicuspid valve (see page 9) dips into the ventricle more deeply than it does in healthy people. Mitral valve prolapse does not usually cause problems. Occasionally, however, the valve can be the site of a blood clot,[8] which can embolize.

Arterial dissection

Violent movements or neck injuries – such as a car accident – can damage the carotid or vertebral arteries. As a result, blood can get inside the layers that make up the wall of the blood vessel (see page 11). This pushes the sides of the vessel together, blocking the blood flow to the brain. In other cases, the damage roughens the smooth inner lining of the vessel, which increases the chance that a clot will form.[8]

Such damage, which doctors call arterial dissection, tends to occur in younger people more than other forms of ischaemic stroke. Traditionally, doctors regarded arterial dissection as relatively uncommon. However, the improved ability to image the neck is increasing the number of people diagnosed with arterial dissection.[5]

Strokes and heart attacks

Up to one person in 20 who has a heart attack also has a stroke. For example, emboli can arise from clots on the dead muscle in the heart. The traditional image of a heart attack is a person clutching their chest and falling down. However, some people – especially the elderly and those with diabetes – can experience relatively painless heart attacks. In such cases, a stroke might be the first sign that they have suffered a heart attack.[8]

The link between strokes and heart attacks runs both ways. If you have atherosclerosis in one part of your body, the chances are that you have plaques elsewhere, including in the vessels supplying your heart. Each year, about one person in 50 who has survived a TIA or stroke experiences a heart attack. People who have other cardiovascular diseases (such as peripheral vascular disease) or diabetes or who have survived a severe stroke are especially likely to have a heart attack.[26]

Peripheral vascular disease

In peripheral vascular disease (also called peripheral arterial disease), atherosclerotic plaques develop in arteries supplying your kidneys, stomach and other organs, and your limbs. For example, the reduced blood supply to your legs – the most common site of peripheral atherosclerosis – can cause intermittent claudication (from the Latin for 'to limp').

People who have intermittent claudication report aching or cramping pain, with tightness or fatigue in their leg muscles or buttocks. Some people find that the pain arises during strenuous activity or when they walk up stairs. People with more severe peripheral vascular disease may develop intermittent claudication after walking only a few metres. The pain subsides after a few minutes' rest. Severe blockages to the blood flow can cause gangrene (tissue death), which may even end in the need for amputation. In other words, don't ignore intermittent claudication – it could be a warning that you may have cardiovascular disease.

Cardiac arrest

During a cardiac arrest, the heart stops pumping and blood no longer reaches the brain. You will lose consciousness almost immediately and won't breathe normally. Several types of event can trigger cardiac arrest, including a heart attack, electrocution, choking, losing large amounts of blood and being very hot or very cold. However, a type of arrhythmia (see page 35) called ventricular fibrillation is the most common cause of cardiac arrest.

During ventricular fibrillation, the ventricles stop pumping. Defibrillators deliver an electric shock through the chest wall, which sometimes restores normal beats. Without cardiopulmonary resuscitation and defibrillation, most cardiac arrests kill. If you think someone is in cardiac arrest, call 999 immediately and give cardiopulmonary resuscitation.

Sickle cell anaemia

As mentioned in Chapter 2, people of African Caribbean descent are more likely than white people to develop a stroke. Several factors contribute to this increased risk, including sickle cell anaemia, a genetic disease that causes crescent-shaped red blood cells (eryth-rocytes). Sickle cell anaemia seems to protect against malaria and is most common in people of African heritage.

The abnormally shaped red blood cells can clump inside blood vessels, which increases the risk of a stroke. As a result, children with sickle cell disease are between 200 and 400 times more likely to have a stroke than those without the condition.[7] About 11 per cent of untreated people with sickle cell disease have a stroke before the age of 20 years. Approximately 24 per cent have a stroke before the age of 45 years.[38] Blood transfusions replace sickle cells with normally shaped erythrocytes and, therefore, cut stroke risk.[7]

Polycythaemia

People with polycythaemia produce too many red blood cells. This thickens the blood, which cannot circulate easily (imagine treacle rather than water). In addition, red blood cells can clump, which blocks small vessels and causes strokes, pulmonary embolism (see page 22) and heart attacks.[8] Regularly removing about a pint of blood and taking drugs to slow down the production of red blood cells can help treat polycythaemia.

Diabetes

Diabetes is a complex disease with a simple cause. Cells are, essentially, biological factories. All factories need fuel: cells use a type of sugar called glucose to generate energy. The body extracts glucose from carbohydrates (such as sugars) that we eat.

A hormone called insulin stimulates cells to take glucose from the blood. Without insulin, most cells cannot use glucose. So, glucose levels in the blood rise in people who do not produce enough insulin. In other people with diabetes, insulin does not work properly when it reaches the cells – so-called insulin resistance (some people have both problems). Again, the cells do not absorb glucose and the amount in the blood rises. These dangerously high blood sugar levels (hyperglycaemia) poison cells, potentially causing debilitating, distressing and disabling complications such as pain, ulcers, amputations, heart disease, blindness and strokes.

Type 1 diabetes

Doctors recognize several types of diabetes, of which type 1 and type 2 are the most common. Normally, our immune system attacks invading pathogens (such as bacteria, viruses and parasites), while limiting 'collateral' damage to healthy tissues. The immune system launches this targeted attack using proteins called antibodies, which identify the invaders and trigger the reactions that destroy the pathogens.

Occasionally, however, the immune system produces antibodies against healthy tissues. Type 1 diabetes, which usually arises in childhood or young adulthood, occurs when the immune system produces antibodies that destroy cells in an organ just under the ribcage, called the pancreas, that produces insulin. People with type 1 diabetes need regular insulin injections to replace the missing hormone.

Type 2 diabetes

According to Diabetes UK, type 2 diabetes accounts for between 85 and 90 per cent of diabetes in the UK. Type 2 diabetes usually occurs in obese and overweight people aged over 40 years. However, doctors are diagnosing type 2 diabetes in increasing numbers of children and teenagers. Excess weight causes about 9 in every 10 cases of type 2 diabetes.

Type 2 diabetes shortens life expectancy by up to ten years, largely because of the dramatically increased risk of stroke and other diseases affecting the heart and blood vessels. People with diabetes are, for instance, roughly twice as likely as other people to have a stroke in the five years after their doctor has diagnosed diabetes. Atherosclerosis is responsible for most of this increased risk.

Diabetes UK's online assessment – <www.riskscore.diabetes.org. uk> – lets you determine how likely you are to develop type 2 diabetes. If you are at high risk, see your doctor. If you are at medium risk, follow the lifestyle advice later in the book to cut your risk of stroke and other diabetic complications. But don't be complacent even if you're at low risk. There are many other ways to suffer a stroke.

Legal and illegal drugs

As mentioned above, smoking and alcohol are among the most important risk factors for stroke. However, a variety of other legal and illegal drugs can also trigger strokes.

Smoking

Quitting smoking is one of the best ways to cut stroke risk. Smoking directly causes almost one in five strokes.[22] For example, researchers combined 81 studies that involved almost 4 million people. Compared to non-smokers, smokers have an increased risk of:

- ischaemic stroke in women by 54 per cent and in men by 53 per cent, and
- haemorrhagic stroke in women by 63 per cent and in men by 22 per cent.[22]

The risk of stroke is even higher among heavy smokers and smokers with hypertension:

- A person smoking 20 cigarettes a day is six times more likely to suffer a stroke than a non-smoker.
- According to the Stroke Association, a smoker with hypertension is five times more likely to have a stroke than a smoker with normal blood pressure.
- A smoker with hypertension is 20 times more likely to have a stroke than a non-smoker with normal blood pressure.

Quitting smoking is tough, although the tips on page 105 should help.

Illicit drugs

In young people under the age of 30 years, illicit drugs – such as cocaine – are a leading cause of strokes. Cocaine, amphetamines, ecstasy and some other drugs can trigger a marked rise in blood pressure inside the head. These sudden increases place the blood vessels under considerable strain and, over time, they may rupture, especially if the person has an aneurysm (see page 25) or another weakness in their cardiovascular system.[8]

For example, researchers told the American Stroke Association's International Conference in 2014 that cocaine increases stroke risk in young adults much more than some other factors, such as diabetes, hypertension and smoking. Users were six to seven times more likely to suffer an ischaemic stroke within 24 hours of using cocaine. In addition, cocaine can trigger dangerous spasms in blood vessels, while ecstasy can trigger a venous sinus thrombus (a blood clot in the veins running from the brain).[7]

If you know someone who abuses illegal drugs, you should gently, non-confrontationally, and without condemning their use, ask them to seek help from their GP or local drug services (details are on the NHS Choices website – <www.nhs.uk>) or to contact the drugs advice service Frank – <www.talktofrank.com>). However, do not assume 'legal highs' are risk-free. Definitive studies have examined relatively few legal highs. In most cases, we simply do not know the risks.

Alcohol abuse

A few years ago, a doctor from a Glasgow hospital told a medical meeting that Friday night was stroke night. The bouts of binge drinking produced a dramatic peak in the number of haemorrhagic strokes admitted to the city's accident and emergency departments. According to the Stroke Association, heavy drinkers are about three times more likely to suffer a stroke than those who drink sensibly.

A very British alcohol unit

In the UK, a 'unit' contains eight grams (or ten millilitres) of alcohol. A standard bottle (750 ml) of 12 per cent wine contains nine units – so there are three units in a large (250 ml) glass of wine. A pint of 5 per cent beer or cider also contains three units – that's 24 grams of alcohol. A US 'drink' (as served in a bar in the States) contains 14 grams of alcohol – just under two British units.

Nevertheless, studies showing that drinking small amounts of alcohol is good for your health regularly capture the headlines. For example, a review of 84 studies found that compared to abstaining:[39]

- drinking 2.5–14.9 grams of alcohol a day *reduces* the risk of having a stroke by 20 per cent and the risk of dying from a stroke by 14 per cent;
- drinking 30–60 grams of alcohol a day *increases* the risk of having a stroke by 15 per cent and the risk of dying from a stroke by 10 per cent;
- drinking more than 60 g daily *increases* the risk of having a stroke by 62 per cent and the risk from dying from a stroke by 44 per cent.

In other words, drinkers need to tread a fine line – it is easy to drink too much. We shall look at how to tell if you are drinking too much and some ways to cut down on page 101.

Stress

Few of us avoid the hassles arising from missed trains, long queues or a demanding boss, partner or child. Unfortunately, stress seems to increase the chance of suffering a stroke – a link starkly illustrated by a UK study looking at people who faced the death of a partner. Compared to similar non-bereaved people, those who lost their partner were 140 per cent more likely to experience a stroke during the first 30 days after their loss. After this, the risk was no higher than among non-bereaved people.[40]

Many people react to a stress by becoming angry. Unfortunately, one study found that the risk of an ischaemic stroke was almost eight-fold higher in the two hours after an angry outburst. Another study reported a less dramatic effect, but the risk was still 66 per cent higher. Anger can also drive blood pressure up. So, an intracranial aneurysm is about six times more likely to burst in the two hours after an angry outburst than at other times.[41]

Depression

Stress contributes to depression – which is more than feeling a bit 'down in the dumps'. It's profound, debilitating mental and physical lethargy, a pervasive sense of worthlessness and intense, deep, unshakable sadness, guilt and self-loathing. If you've never experienced depression, it's difficult to appreciate how devastating the condition is.

As we shall see later, stroke seems to increase the risk of depression, as a reaction to the life-changing event and because of damage to parts of the brain that regulate emotion (see page 122). However, the relationship between depression and stroke runs both ways: depression seems to increase the risk of suffering a stroke by about 34 per cent. Depression also increases the risk of developing heart disease (by 81 per cent), diabetes (by 60 per cent), obesity (by 58 per cent) and hypertension (by 42 per cent).

Several factors may link depression to stroke and the other conditions. For example, depressed people are less likely to eat a healthy diet – which helps fuel the increase in diabetes, obesity and hypertension. Depressed people are also more likely to smoke and abuse alcohol and illicit drugs. In many cases, drug abuse seems to be an attempt, albeit dangerous, at self-medication to alleviate the burden imposed by depression. Chapter 7 looks at the intimate link between depression and stroke.

Shingles and other infections

Several infections seem to increase the risk of stroke including syphilis, HIV[7] and, more commonly, shingles and influenza. For example, strokes are more common during the winter, partly because influenza is more widespread than in the summer.[31]

The varicella-zoster virus (VZV) causes chickenpox, which most of us catch during childhood. VZV also causes shingles (also known as herpes zoster; a different virus causes genital herpes). After you recover from chickenpox, VZV can 'hide' in nerves. Later in life, physical and emotional stress, some medicines, age and so on can reactivate VZV, which moves along the nerves into the skin, where it causes the characteristic rash of shingles.[42] Occasionally, VZV moves along the nerves to parts of the head where its re-emergence can trigger TIAs and strokes.

A study from the UK followed 106,601 people with herpes zoster and 213,202 controls without the infection for, on average, just over six years. After adjusting for other risk factors, people with herpes zoster were 15 per cent more likely to have a TIA and 10 per cent more likely to have a heart attack. Overall, herpes zoster did not increase stroke risk. However, patients who developed herpes zoster between the ages of 18 and 40 years of age were 142 per cent more likely to have a TIA, while the risk of a stroke or heart attack increased by 74 and 49 per cent, respectively.[42]

Another study of 6,584 patients, again from the UK, reported that the risk of stroke was 63 per cent higher in the first four weeks after doctors diagnosed herpes zoster. The risk declined to a 42 per cent increased risk during five to 12 weeks later, and to a 23 per cent increased risk during weeks 13 to 26. No link between herpes zoster persisted after this. People who developed herpes ophthalmicus, where the shingles rash arises around the eye, showed a stronger link – rising to a 238 per cent increase in stroke risk during weeks five to 12 after diagnosis, and then declining. Antiviral medications reduced the stroke risk to around 20 per cent overall and reduced the peak risk with herpes ophthalmicus to 157 per cent.[43] In other words, see your doctor if you develop a rash.

Risk factors for women

Women share many risk factors for stroke – such as hypertension, smoking and high cholesterol – with men. However, some risks are unique to women, reflecting the influence of female hormones, pregnancy and childbirth. For example, women who develop pre-eclampsia (dangerously increased blood pressure and high levels of protein in urine during pregnancy) are twice as likely to have a stroke and four times more likely to develop hypertension in later life than mothers-to-be those whose blood pressure remains normal during pregnancy. This section looks at some stroke risk factors that are especially or exclusively hazardous for women.

Oral contraceptives

Oral contraceptives increase the risk of hypertension and stroke. When researchers looked at 50 studies, they found no evidence that oral contraceptives increased the risk of haemorrhagic strokes or heart attacks. However, oral contraceptives almost trebled the risk of venous thromboembolism (a blood clot in a vein) and roughly doubled the risk of ischaemic stroke.[44]

Despite the increased risk, very few women have a stroke solely because they take oral contraceptives. According to the UK guidelines, the pill causes one extra ischaemic stroke per year for every 20,000 women using low-dose oestrogen oral contraception[5] – that's the same as one person in about 40 jumbo jets full of people. In general, oral contraceptives or hormone replacement therapy increases stroke risk only in women with other risk factors, such as migraines (see below) or hypertension.[3] If you have other risk factors or a history of TIA or stroke, discuss other hormonal and non-hormonal contraceptives with your doctor or nurse.

Migraines with aura

Sometimes it's easy to confuse a migraine with a stroke. Some strokes begin with an aura, which neurologist Stephen Siberstein describes as 'shimmering, flashing, weird perceptions' that 'seem inexplicable, even frightening'. Some people report blindness – a missing area in their field of vision – as well as dizziness, numbness and tingling.[45]

Migraines are common: about 11 per cent of adults experience these headaches, which typically emerge over several minutes.[8,45] Many people can predict that migraine is on the way: they may experience an aura, feel nauseous or 'just know', although they cannot put their finger on why.[8] Strokes, in contrast, tend to emerge rapidly, often within seconds and without warning.

Women are four times more likely to suffer from migraines with aura than men. In one study of almost 28,000 women aged at least 45 years, those who experienced migraine with aura were around twice as likely to have an ischaemic stroke during the ten-year investigation as those without migraines.[46] The reason why the women in the study were at increased risk is not clear. However, women who experience migraines with aura seem to be about twice as likely to experience several other cardiovascular problems including heart attacks, angina and needing surgery to open blocked vessels.[46] So, an underlying abnormality in the blood vessels may contribute to cardiovascular disease and migraines.

Atrial fibrillation

When researchers combined 17 studies, women with atrial fibrillation (see page 35) were 31 per cent more likely to have a stroke than men with the arrhythmia. Women with atrial fibrillation who were taking oral anticoagulants (see page 55) were especially likely to have a stroke – a 49 per cent increase compared to men – than in those not receiving drugs to prevent clots (29 per cent).[47]

Strokes during pregnancy

Strokes during pregnancy are 'infrequent but often catastrophic'.[28] For instance, strokes account for between 12 and 14 per cent of maternal deaths and are the most common cause of death in mothers who develop eclampsia (seizures during pregnancy). Between 13 and 35 per cent of mothers who experience a subarachnoid haemorrhage during pregnancy die. Foetal mortality after the mother has a subarachnoid haemorrhage is between 7 and 25 per cent. Overall, pregnancy increases the risk of a stroke by up to 13 times.[28]

The timing of pregnancy-related strokes

About 11 per cent of pregnancy-related strokes occur while the mother is expecting. Approximately 41 per cent occur immediately around labour and during delivery. The remaining 48 per cent occur in the six weeks after birth.[28] The risk of subarachnoid haemorrhage increases as pregnancy progresses. A third of pregnancy-related subarachnoid haemorrhages occur in the second trimester and more than half during the third trimester.[28]

Most strokes in mothers-to-be occur because pregnancy exacerbates one or more existing risk factors.[7] However, strokes can also occur because of the dramatic changes to the body during pregnancy.[28]

The amniotic fluid, which bathes and cushions the baby in the womb, can trigger an embolism, for example.[7] Indeed, numerous factors make a stroke during pregnancy more likely, including:

- Advancing age – older women are more likely to have a pregnancy-related stroke. Compared to women aged under 20 years, mothers between 35 and 39 years of age are 90 per cent more likely to have a pregnancy-related stroke, and those aged 40 years or older are 230 per cent more likely.[28]
- Hypertension before pregnancy – women who had hypertension before they became pregnant are about 2.6 times more likely to experience a pregnancy-related stroke than those who had normal blood pressure. Developing hypertension during pregnancy increases the risk to a similar extent (2.4 times).[28]
- Pre-eclampsia or eclampsia – these conditions increase stroke risk about 10 times compared to those without the condition.[28]
- Cocaine, amphetamine and tobacco use – using these substances while expecting a baby roughly doubles the risk of pregnancy-related stroke.[28] Taking drugs is incredibly dangerous for the baby in numerous other ways. If you fall pregnant when misusing legal drugs (including tobacco and alcohol) or illicit drugs you must talk to your GP or a drug and alcohol service as soon as possible.
- Migraines – women who experience migraines are almost 17 times more likely to experience a pregnancy-related stroke.[28]
- Sickle cell disease (see page 38) – women with sickle cell disease are almost nine times more likely to experience a pregnancy-related stroke than those without this condition.[28]
- Thrombocytopenia – women with thrombocytopenia are about six times more likely to experience a stroke during pregnancy.[28] People with thrombocytopenia have low levels of platelets (see page 55). This means that their blood does not clot properly.

Risk factors come to the fore

As mentioned above, underlying risk factors for stroke seem to come to the fore during pregnancy. A strong family history of heart disease or stroke roughly trebles the risk of pre-eclampsia, for example.[28] Furthermore, women who develop gestational hypertension, pre-eclampsia and other complications of pregnancy associated with hypertension are between two and four times more likely than other women to have cardiovascular disease, thrombo-embolism or stroke in later life.[28] This suggests that many women who experience strokes during pregnancy have a predisposition to cardiovascular disease.

In addition, clots in the cerebral veins and sinuses are more common in women than men. In women, these clots usually develop during late pregnancy or soon after birth. The major veins in the brain contain folds called sinuses, which lack muscle and so cannot contract to push the blood along. Blood can pool in these sinuses. In turn, the blood may clot, which reduces flow away from the brain. This means the pressure inside the blood vessels can rise, parts of the brain may swell and bleed, and areas can become ischaemic.[28] Pregnant women who experience persistent headaches should see a doctor. However, at least 90 per cent of mothers survive thrombosis in the cerebral veins and sinuses and few develop persistent mental or physical disabilities.

4

Treating stroke

If I'd like you to remember one thing from this book, it is to seek medical attention as soon as you experience a symptom that might indicate a stroke (see page ix). Modern treatments, especially when used quickly, dramatically increase your chances of surviving a stroke and protect against serious disability.

Nevertheless, diagnosing stroke is not always easy. Several illnesses (including epilepsy, brain tumours and multiple sclerosis) can mimic strokes.[7] Haemorrhagic and ischaemic strokes can cause the same symptoms. However, doctors need to get the diagnosis right. Some drugs – such as anticoagulants and aspirin (see page 55) – that can save lives in people with ischaemic strokes can cause potentially deadly brain haemorrhages in susceptible people. Yet even today, about a fifth of stroke diagnoses made in a typical accident and emergency department are wrong.[7]

Advances in treatment

Stroke treatments have come a long way in the last few hundred years. In the sixteenth century, healers suggested that stroke survivors should drink cinnamon water. It probably didn't help, but cinnamon water was more pleasant and less harmful than the treatments proposed by some physicians in the eighteenth century, who linked stroke to eating 'large, indigestible' meals. They recommended a 'stimulating vomit' and 'a warm cordial purge'. A leading medical textbook published in 1812 advocated 'speedy bloodletting', which physicians regarded as 'often of considerable importance' for 'sudden attacks of apoplexy'.[48] Bloodletting, vomits, purges and 'stimulating' enemas remained popular stroke treatments, at least among doctors if not their patients, until the beginning of the twentieth century.[21]

Brain scans

Until the 1970s, doctors had to guess the cause of a stroke, which was often extremely difficult. If atherosclerosis has narrowed the carotid artery, doctors can sometimes hear a whooshing sound (called a bruit) by using a stethoscope placed on the person's neck. But bruits are not particularly reliable.

The introduction of computed tomography (CT), previously called computerized axial tomography (CAT) scans, in the 1970s revolutionized diagnosis.[7] For the first time, doctors could look inside the brain of a living person to identify the type of stroke and so could target treatment with unprecedented accuracy. Doctors also realized that some people had micro-bleeds that caused silent – often lacunar – strokes that did not cause noticeable symptoms.

Almost all stroke patients have a brain scan while in hospital, although not always within the recommended 24 hours.[5] Brain scans can, for example, help doctors decide whether an ischaemic stroke, a haemorrhagic stroke or some other condition caused your symptoms.[7,20] However, about one person in a hundred develops massive bleeding after an ischaemic stroke. This can resemble a haemorrhagic stroke on brain scans. So, the earlier the hospital performs the scan, the better.[7]

In some cases, doctors may use ultrasound scans or a Doppler scan to investigate the carotid artery. A Doppler scan measures the speed at which blood cells move along the vessel. The speed changes if the artery narrows. A transcranial Doppler scan can help indicate the health of the main arteries that supply the brain.[8] Your doctor might also suggest cerebral angiography. The surgeon moves a thin tube called a catheter to the opening of the neck arteries and then injects a dye. This shows up all the arteries in the neck on X-ray.

A doctor or nurse will also take a blood sample, which will be used to check for, for example:

- the number of red blood cells – for example, people with poly-cythaemia produce too many red blood cells (see page 50);
- how long your blood takes to clot – people whose blood does not clot effectively may be at increased risk of haemorrhagic strokes;
- your blood glucose level – very low levels can cause symptoms that mimic strokes.

These insights help rule out other causes for your symptoms.

The benefits of a stroke unit

A stroke unit covers a specific geographical area and employs a co-ordinated, multidisciplinary team that is experienced in stroke care and rehabilitation. Care from a specialized stroke team improves your physical and psychological performance, shortens hospital stay, reduces the likelihood that you will need care in a nursing home and cuts deaths by up to 28 per cent.[20] Several factors contribute to this improved performance. For example, people on stroke units usually have more contact with staff and spend less time in bed.[49]

Clot-busting drugs

People with ischaemic strokes often receive a thrombolytic drug, which breaks down the clot that blocks the artery after an embolism or when an atherosclerotic plaque ruptures. Rapid treatment with a thrombolytic drug restores blood flow to the brain, which limits further damage caused by an ischaemic stroke. So, the sooner treatment restores blood flow, the better your chances of surviving and the less damage your brain endures.[23]

Indeed, each minute saved between the start of symptoms and treatment may preserve two million brain cells and 14 billion synapses, the junctions between nerve cells.[50,51] To look at it another way: each hour a stroke remains untreated, the brain ages by 3.6 years.[51] Against this background, thrombolysis with a drug called tissue-type plasminogen activator (tPA) more than doubles the likelihood that the survivor will recover without disability, provided treatment starts within 1.5 hours of the onset of symptoms. Starting tPA between 3 and 4.5 hours after symptoms start increases the chance of disability-free recovery by 30 per cent.[50] That is why it is so important to call 999 if you or someone around you shows stroke signs (see page ix).

On the other hand, thrombolysis makes it harder for your blood to clot. This means that the risk of fatal and non-fatal intracerebral haemorrhages rises within seven days of treatment.[5] In most cases, the benefits outweigh the risks. But speak to the stroke team if you or your carer is worried.

Sometimes surgeons use a mechanical 'clot retrieval system' to remove the blockage by passing a catheter into the top of the leg and into the cerebral blood vessels. However, the risk of bleeding seems to be similar to thrombolysis.[7]

Anticoagulation

DVTs (see page 22) are common among stroke survivors. Scans of the legs and pelvis performed three weeks after an ischaemic stroke found DVTs in 40 per cent of survivors. Furthermore, 12 per cent had pulmonary embolisms.[26] Other studies suggest that up to 50 per cent of people with hemiplegia (weakness or paralysis on one side of the body) develop DVT after a stroke, with between 1 per cent and 7 per cent experiencing pulmonary embolism.[3] While the figures vary depending on the detection method and the patients studied, DVT is clearly a common and potentially serious problem for stroke survivors.

Pulmonary embolisms generally occur between two and four weeks after the stroke. However, cognitive problems, speech impair-

Compression stockings and intermittent pneumatic compression

Although widely used to prevent DVTs in other circumstances, doctors advise against compression stocking after strokes. One study, for example, found that compression stockings did not reduce the risk of DVT, pulmonary embolism or death. However, the stockings made skin ulcers four times more likely and might reduce blood flow to the feet.[26]

In contrast, intermittent pneumatic compression (IPC) dramatically reduces DVT risk. IPC uses inflatable sleeves wrapped around the legs. A timer inflates these automatically, one side at a time, to compress the legs at set intervals, such as after the veins refill with blood.

The CLOTS-3 study, for example, used IPC in 1,438 patients who could not walk to the toilet unaided after suffering a stroke. Treatment lasted an average of 12.5 days. Another 1,438 immobile patients – called the control group – did not receive IPC. Over the 30 days after the start of compression, about 9 per cent per cent of the IPC group and 12 per cent of the control group developed a DVT. In other words, IPC reduced the risk of DVT by 35 per cent.[52]

ment, reduced consciousness, pneumonia and the fever that can follow a stroke can make diagnosis difficult. For example, DVTs cause a swollen, hot or painful limb, as well as fever.[3] But up to 60 per cent of people develop a fever in the 72 hours after experiencing an ischaemic stroke. This may arise because of the stress on the body caused by the stroke, an infection, or following damage to the part of the brain that keeps our body temperature constant. Unfortunately, fever can exacerbate the damage by increasing the demand on the injured brain cells.[26] Heparin can reduce the risk of DVTs and pulmonary emboli.

Heparin

During the First World War, researchers in the USA isolated heparin from liver – *hepra* is Greek for 'liver'.[53] Today, heparin – one of the oldest drugs that doctors still commonly prescribe – keeps blood clots from expanding or travelling to another part of your body.

Doctors call the original version of heparin 'unfractionated' heparin. Although unfractionated heparin is highly effective, users often need regular, time-consuming monitoring and, in many cases, frequent dose changes. Unfractionated heparin can also cause thrombocytopenia (abnormally low platelet numbers), bleeding problems and osteoporosis (brittle bone disease) during long-term use.

These limitations prompted the development of low molecular weight heparins (LMWHs). The manufacturer uses chemicals or enzymes to break the heparin chain, producing fragments that are around a third of the size of the unfractionated version. LMWHs produce a more predictable response and require less intensive monitoring. LMWHs may also be less likely to cause bleeding, thrombocytopenia and osteoporosis than full-sized heparin.

Warfarin

Atrial fibrillation is an important and increasingly common cause of stroke (see page 35). Fortunately, doctors can use several treatments to reduce the risk. For example, beta-blockers, calcium channel blockers and digoxin can slow the racing heart. In addition, several drugs, including warfarin, reduce the risk of blood clots.

Winters are always tough on the herds of cattle in North Dakota, USA and Alberta, Canada. But during the winter of 1921–1922, more than the expected number of cattle died. Some cattle bled to death within a few hours of dehorning. Others died from internal bleeding. A Canadian biologist linked the deaths to sweet clovers that had turned mouldy and that the farmers had used to feed the cattle. Researchers isolated the chemical responsible, which they called dicumarol.[53]

The researchers tried dicumarol as an anticoagulant and as a rat poison. Dicumarol acted too slowly, but a chemical variation – called warfarin – became the most successful rat poison and the most widely used oral anticoagulant.[53] Warfarin can reduce the risk of a stroke by 60 per cent in people with atrial fibrillation, for example.[7] Warfarin and related drugs, called coumarins, interfere with the production of vitamin K, which is needed to clot blood.

Taking a rat poison might seem a strange way to remain healthy. However, warfarin illustrates a basic principle of medicine: the dose and use distinguish medicines from poisons. Even drinking too much water can kill. In 2007, a woman died after drinking six litres of water in three hours. Botulinum toxin, produced by a bacterium, is one of the most deadly poisons. However, minuscule doses can alleviate muscle spasms and spasticity (see page 79) in stroke survivors and reduce the appearance of wrinkles.

As you might expect, uncontrolled bleeding – including intracerebral bleeds – is warfarin's main side effect. In any year, about 5 per cent of people taking warfarin have a minor bleed, while 1 per cent have a serious haemorrhage.[8] In addition, warfarin can interact with many other drugs to increase the risk of side effects. So, it is important to tell your doctor and pharmacist about any other drugs you are taking. You will also need regular tests to see how long your blood takes to clot. This allows the doctor to ensure that the dose of warfarin is right for your needs.

NICE now recommends anticoagulation with one of the newer drugs (such as apixaban, dabigatran etexilate or rivaroxaban) or with a vitamin K antagonist (such as warfarin) for atrial fibrillation. Some of the newer drugs act more quickly than warfarin, have fewer interactions with other drugs and foods, and do not require intensive monitoring.[5] However, doctors cannot reverse excessive anticoagulation by adding vitamin K, as you can with warfarin. Your doctor should discuss which anticoagulant is best for you.

Aspirin

When the German pharmaceutical company Bayer launched aspirin in the 1890s, doctors worried that the drug could harm the heart. Bayer even labelled the bottles, 'Aspirin does not affect the heart'. Today, we know that aspirin does affect the heart – but in a beneficial way.[53] When you start bleeding, platelets gather at the wound and stick together forming a clot. Aspirin prevents this 'platelet aggregation'. So, aspirin helps prevent the clots that lead to emboli and those that form when an atherosclerotic plaque ruptures, reducing the risk of a heart attack or stroke.

However, because aspirin reduces your blood's ability to clot, before you start taking aspirin your doctor will make sure (using a brain scan) that an intracerebral haemorrhage has *not* caused your symptoms.[3] And you should never take aspirin – to relieve a headache, for example – if you're using other anticoagulants unless your doctor suggests the combination. You could risk excessive bleeding and even a haemorrhagic stroke.

Aspirin, long a mainstay of medicine boxes, is highly effective. For example, about one extra person remains independent after a stroke for every 100 who take aspirin in the first two weeks after a stroke. Aspirin has the same benefit over the next 50 weeks.[7] In people at high risk (for example, following a heart attack or stroke), aspirin reduces the likelihood of stroke, heart attack or death from vascular disease by 23 per cent. Similarly, in people who have already had a stroke, aspirin reduces the chance of a recurrence by about 15 per cent.[25] You will probably take 300 mg of aspirin as soon as possible after the doctor or paramedic suspects an ischaemic stroke.[20] Longer-term, your doctor may reduce the dose, but never change or stop taking your medicines without speaking to your doctor first.

More recently, pharmaceutical companies introduced several other drugs (such as dipyridamole and clopidogrel) that also target platelets. These may have advantages over aspirin in some people. A study called the Antithrombotic Trialists' Collaboration showed that in people who had suffered a stroke or TIA, antiplatelet drugs reduced the risk of a heart attack or a stroke or of dying from cardiovascular disease by 22 per cent.[5]

Clopidogrel used alone is as effective as the combination of aspirin plus dipyridamole. Both seem to be more effective than aspirin used alone. Clopidogrel and the combination both prevent about one additional cardiovascular event for every 100 patients treated for a year compared to aspirin alone.[5] This means that 99 people do not benefit, but are at risk of side effects.

However, as the adverse effects differ, you can switch antiplatelet drugs if you develop side effects. Aspirin, for instance, causes side effects that include upset stomach, indigestion, bruising and bleeding in the stomach. Dipyridamole can cause, among other reactions, diarrhoea, dizziness, nausea, dyspepsia, headache and muscle aches. Clopidogrel can cause diarrhoea and a skin rash and bleeding.[7,8] So, it is important to discuss the risks and benefits of each antiplatelet drug with your doctor.

Hypertension

Hypertension (dangerously high blood pressure) is one of the most important risk factors for strokes. For example, a study called PROGRESS included 6105 people. Of these, 52 per cent did not have hypertension at the start of the four-year study. Nevertheless, reducing blood pressure by 12/5 mmHg (see page 26) reduced the risk of recurrent stroke by 43 per cent and major coronary events (such as heart attacks) by 35 per cent compared to an inactive placebo.[5,54]

The UK's stroke guidelines suggest that most people who survived a stroke or TIA should have a blood pressure below 130/80 mmHg.[5] So, if a doctor or nurse has not taken your blood pressure for a few months, speak to your GP. You can use a combination of lifestyle changes and drugs to bring your pressure back to safe levels.

Don't underestimate the effectiveness of lifestyle changes. In most people, 'realistic changes in diet and lifestyle' reduce diastolic blood pressure by 2–3 mmHg.[55] However, some people do much better than this – especially when they combine several changes (see Table 4.1). Nevertheless, most people also need to take blood pressure-lowering drugs (antihypertensives). Taken regularly, depending on the drug and dose, antihypertensives reduce the risk of:

- stroke by 20–39 per cent;
- coronary heart disease by 19–20 per cent; and
- major cardiovascular events (stroke, heart attack, heart failure or death from any cardiovascular cause) by 15–28 per cent.[56]

Table 4.1 Lifestyle changes' impact on blood pressure

Lifestyle change	Reduction in systolic blood pressure
Maintaining body mass index (BMI; see page 109) between 20 and 25 kg/m²	5–10 mmHg per 10 kg weight loss
Eating a diet rich in fruit, vegetables and low-fat dairy products, and low in saturated and total fat	8–14 mmHg
Reducing salt consumption to less than 2.4 grams of sodium (less than six grams of salt)	2–8 mmHg
Taking regular aerobic activity (e.g. brisk walking for at least 30 minutes a day)	4–9 mmHg
Limiting alcohol consumption to 21 units a week or less (for men) or 14 units a week or less (for women)	2–4 mmHg

Adapted from Williams et al.[57]

Overall, a 10 mmHg reduction in systolic blood pressure reduces stroke risk by 41 per cent and ischaemic heart disease by 22 per cent.[1]

Lowering blood pressure immediately after a stroke

Blood pressure is often high immediately after a stroke because of the stroke itself, anxiety or because the person already had hypertension. However, doctors worry that lowering the pressure may reduce the amount of blood reaching the brain and, therefore, worsen the damage. As a result, doctors generally treat raised blood pressure after a stroke only if the person is at marked risk of further complications. In general, blood pressure tends to decline in the two weeks after a stroke.[20] After this, your GP or another doctor should assess whether you need to make lifestyle changes and take drugs to tackle hypertension.

Doctors can choose from among a wide range of antihypertensives, including angiotensin-converting enzyme (ACE) inhibitors, diuretics, beta-blockers and calcium channel blockers. There's not space here to discuss the pros and cons of each. So, talk to your doctor and check out NHS Choices and patient groups' websites. This therapeutic diversity means, for example, if you suffer, or are at risk of, a side effect – such as asthma with beta-blockers, a persistent dry cough with ACE inhibitors, increases in sugar levels in your blood with some diuretics, or flushed face or headaches with calcium channel blockers – doctors can usually find an alternative.

Unfortunately, a single antihypertensive controls blood pressure adequately in only 20–30 per cent of patients.[58] Most people need at least two antihypertensives that work in different ways: such as a diuretic and an ACE inhibitor. Many people need at least three. That's one reason why it's so important to change your lifestyle: you may be less likely to need multiple drugs. Lifestyle modification can lower blood pressure as much as a single antihypertensive.[57]

Cholesterol-lowering drugs

Medicine usually advances in small steps. Occasionally, however, a study is so important that treatment changes almost overnight. In the early 1990s, doctors knew that cholesterol filled atherosclerotic plaques. However, there was no firm evidence that cutting blood cholesterol levels saved lives. Then, in 1994, *The Lancet* reported results from the Scandinavian Simvastatin Survival Study (4S).[59]

The 4S study included 4,444 people with raised serum cholesterol who had angina (chest pains on exercise, usually caused by atherosclerosis) or had previously suffered a heart attack. All those in the study ate a low-fat diet and received simvastatin, a cholesterol-lowering drug, or placebo. After, on average, almost five and a half years, simvastatin reduced total cholesterol by 25 per cent, cut LDL by 35 per cent and increased HDL levels by 8 per cent. Deaths overall fell by 30 per cent, while deaths from heart disease declined by 42 per cent. The number of people who experienced at least one major coronary event declined by 34 per cent.[59] Since 4S, numerous studies confirmed that cholesterol-lowering drugs – several related medicines followed in the wake of simvastatin, collectively called statins – improve cholesterol levels in the blood and, therefore, protect against stroke.

The Heart Protection Study, for instance, reported that in people at high risk of a cardiovascular event, simvastatin taken daily reduced the risk of vascular deaths by 17 per cent, stroke by 25 per cent and major coronary events by 27 per cent. Another study (called SPARCL) investigated atorvastatin (another statin) in people who had survived a TIA or stroke in the previous 6 months. Atorvastatin reduced the risk of another stroke by 15 per cent and major coronary events by 35 per cent.[5] Overall, a reduction in LDL of 1.0 millimoles per litre seems to reduce the risk of any stroke by 17 per cent and ischaemic strokes by 19 per cent. (However, these are averages and your response may differ.) Statins also seem to slow or, in some cases, possibly reverse atherosclerosis.[3]

However, some studies suggest that statins may increase the risk of haemorrhagic stroke. As a result, doctors tend to be cautious when prescribing statins to patients who had an intracerebral haemorrhage.[5] In addition, statins can cause several side effects, including:

- headache;
- dizziness;
- changes in the enzymes produced by your liver;
- rash;
- myalgia (muscle pain and cramps); and
- rhabdomyolysis, in which muscle damage releases a protein called myoglobin into the blood stream – excessive levels of myoglobin can lead to kidney damage.

The Medicines and Healthcare products Regulatory Agency (MHRA), which controls drugs in the UK, recently examined the evidence regarding the safety of statins. The MHRA confirmed that the 'benefits continue to outweigh the risks of any side effects'. Mild, muscle-related problems are the most frequently reported side effects with statins. However, the MHRA estimate that a person would have to take a statin for, on average, 526 years before experiencing muscle pain (190 cases per 100,000 patient years) and 62,500 years to get rhabdomyolysis (1.6 per 100,000 patient years). But if you feel unwell while taking statins, see your GP.

Keep taking the treatment

Despite reducing the risk of a stroke and other cardiovascular diseases, many survivors do not take their medication as recommended. Cognitive impairment may mean that a survivor simply forgets. Problems with dexterity or swallowing can make taking medicines difficult. Adherence may pose a particular problem for younger people as they may feel that taking medicines disrupts their lifestyle.

Sticking to a routine can help. Some people leave their medicine where they can see it (such as on the breakfast table).[6] Your pharmacist and rehabilitation team can offer aids such as large-print labels, bottles with non-childproof tops, and 'dosette' boxes that allow you to divide treatment by time and day over a week.[5] A doctor may be able to suggest an alternative drug that means taking medication less frequently if you find the regimen disrupts your lifestyle excessively. So, it is important to admit that you have an issue to your GP, nurse or pharmacist. It could save your life.

Surgery for strokes

As mentioned above, surgery to stop the bleeding, relieve the pressure and bypass the burst blood vessel is often the only treatment for haemorrhagic stroke.[15,20] So patients who the accident and emergency team suspect of having a haemorrhagic stroke need to see a neurosurgeon as soon as possible after being admitted to hospital with a stroke. Neurosurgeons can confirm the diagnosis and assess whether patients who have suffered a haemorrhagic stroke need an operation to avoid another bleed.[20] Several other operations can reduce the risk of stroke in other circumstances, as discussed below. However, strokes can arise during surgery, including some operations for heart disease.[7,60] So, discuss the risks and benefits of any operation fully with the surgeon.

Carotid endarterectomy

The gradual development of atherosclerotic plaques can narrow carotid arteries, increasing the risk that they will burst, trigger a clot and lead to another TIA or stroke. An operation called a carotid endarterectomy widens your carotid artery.

A carotid endarterectomy usually takes one to two hours under a general or local anaesthetic. The surgeon makes a small cut into your neck. In some cases, the surgeon uses a small plastic tube, called a shunt, to divert blood around the operation site. The surgeon removes the inner lining of the narrowed part of the artery along with any plaque. The surgeon then closes the cut with stitches or a special patch.

The effectiveness of an endarterectomy depends on how soon the surgeon performs the operation. If performed within two weeks of a minor stroke or TIA, a carotid endarterectomy reduces the risk of stroke recurrence in people with at least 50 per cent stenosis (in other words, the plaque blocks half the vessel). Operating on seven people with 50–69 per cent stenosis within two weeks of the TIA or minor stroke will prevent one stroke. Operating on three people with at least 70 per cent stenosis within two weeks of the TIA or minor stroke will prevent one stroke.[3] However, six and two people, respectively, do not benefit from the operation. However, they are still at risk of complications (see below).

Two weeks after the TIA or minor stroke, endarterectomy benefits only those people with at least 70 per cent stenosis. For example:[3]

- Six operations are needed to prevent one stroke in people with at least 70 per cent stenosis performed between two and four weeks after the TIA or minor stroke.
- Nine operations are needed to prevent one stroke when performed between four and 12 weeks after the TIA or minor stroke.
- More than 12 weeks after the TIA or minor stroke, endarterectomy is no longer effective.

The effectiveness of an endarterectomy also depends on the degree of stenosis. For example, a study of 6,092 patients found that carotid endarterectomy reduced the risk of ischaemic stroke on the side of the brain that the surgeon operated on by:

- 16 per cent over the next five years in patients with 70–99 per cent stenosis;
- almost 5 per cent in patients with 50–69 per cent stenosis.

Endarterectomy did not seem to benefit people with 30–49 per cent stenosis, and it *increased* the risk of stroke in those with less than 30 per cent stenosis.[5]

Overall, 7 per cent of patients either experienced a stroke or died within 30 days of endarterectomy. The risk of stroke or death may be higher in some people. For example, 11 per cent of those with crescendo TIA (see page 16) die in the 30 days after the operation.[5]

You and your family need to understand fully the risks and benefits and discuss them with your doctor.

Angioplasty and stents

Another approach uses a wire-mesh tube called a stent to open the artery. The surgeon threads a catheter tipped with a balloon and guided by X-ray to the blockage. Once in place, the surgeon inflates the balloon, which compresses the plaque, widens the artery and improves blood flow – a process called angioplasty.

In some cases, the surgeon slips a 'collapsed' stent over the catheter and moves the tube next to the blockage. When the surgeon re-inflates the balloon, the stent expands. The stent remains in place after the balloon deflates. Within a few weeks, the artery's inner lining covers the stent, allowing blood to flow easily without clotting. However, stenting does not seem to be as effective as carotid endarterectomy.[7]

Treating aneurysms

As mentioned before, only about half of people who experience a subarachnoid haemorrhage survive. However, survival increases to 85 per cent among people with a confirmed aneurysm who are managed in a neurosurgical unit. In part, the improved prospects reflect specialist surgeons' ability to repair the weakened and ruptured areas. As mentioned before, surgeons may also suggest reinforcing damaged areas to prevent a stroke from occurring in the first place.

However, deciding when to repair the aneurysm after a stroke can prove difficult. When an aneurysm bursts, the muscles in the blood vessels can go into spasm. This spasm, which usually occurs between three and five days after the stroke, narrows the vessel and can further reduce the blood flow to the brain, which can cause further complications.[8]

Surgeons need to decide whether to operate before the spasms have time to develop or to wait a few weeks for the spasms to subside. You tend to do better if you undergo an operation before the spasms develop. However, these 'early' operations are more likely to cause more complications.[8] If possible, you or your next-of-kin should discuss the risks and benefits with your surgeon.

Decompression surgery

Some large ischaemic strokes in the middle cerebral artery (MCA) can cause swelling over a third of the brain, a condition called malignant MCA syndrome. Up to 80 per cent of people with malignant MCA syndrome die. So, surgeons may remove part of the skull to relieve the pressure and reduce the risk of brain damage. It sounds crude. However, the approach halves the number of deaths and increases the number of people who survive with mild or moderate, rather than severe, disability.[3,7]

If the worst happens

Despite medical, surgical and imaging advances, stroke remains the fourth most common cause of death in the UK. Around 12 per cent of people who have a stroke die during the following week. The stroke itself causes most deaths in the first few days. After this, complications – such as pneumonia or pulmonary embolism – become the main causes of death.[3] As a result, many people need palliative care to alleviate distressing end-of-life symptoms including pain, depression, confusion, agitation, malnutrition and dehydration.[5]

A survey of the relatives of 229 people who died from stroke highlighted the range of possible symptoms that people experienced towards the end of their life. For example:[61]

- Seventy-eight per cent had suffered pain for more than six months during the last year of life. Of those that endured pain in the last year, 43 per cent found the pain 'very distressing'. Inform one of the medical team, if you think your loved one is in pain or expressing distress from any other symptom, whether or not he or she is at the end of life.
- Seventy-eight per cent reported feeling low or miserable for more than six months in the last year of life. Forty-five per cent found the low mood 'very distressing'.

Other common symptoms in the last year of life included:

- urinary incontinence (56 per cent);
- mental confusion (50 per cent);
- constipation (45 per cent);
- breathlessness (37 per cent); and

- faecal incontinence (37 per cent).

Palliative care means focusing on more than the physical symptoms alone. The World Health Organization stresses that palliative medicine should also encompass psychosocial and spiritual care.[62] For instance, spiritual beliefs may influence the choice of treatment for pain and other physical symptoms. (Some people want to go gently into that good night fully aware. Opiates, used as painkillers, can cause mental cloudiness.)

Because the end of life is deeply personal, doctors and nurses individualize palliative care. If a loved one is dying, and is aware enough to speak, gently ask for his or her preferences. If you find this difficult, a doctor or counsellor might help.

The stages of dying

Psychiatrist Elisabeth Kübler-Ross developed the now widely accepted view of grief or catastrophic personal loss, including divorce, unemployment, imprisonment, and suffering a devastating health problem such as a stroke. Survivors and their families tend to pass through five emotional stages:

- denial and isolation – a common initial response to bad news;
- anger – patients ask, 'Why me?' Partners and other carers often bear the brunt of this anger;
- bargaining – patients try to postpone or delay the event, perhaps by prayer or a secret pact with God;
- depression – this can emerge as a 'reaction' to the grief and loss, as a reaction to treatment and physical problems, and as a direct effect of the stroke (see Chapter 7);
- acceptance – the person reaches peace, and some patients and their carers are even able to find 'meaning' in their illness and use the disease as an impetus towards spiritual growth.

The order varies from person to person. You may experience more than one stage at a time. And you may move to and fro between stages.

Helping those left behind

The death of a loved one can prove especially difficult practically, psychologically, spiritually and emotionally. You obviously miss a loved one. However, grief can be profound even if the relationship was difficult: you may grieve for the relationship you never had and now never can.

If someone is dying from the stroke or a complication (such as an infection), you might want to make the most of the time left. However, you might find that your loved one becomes withdrawn. A severe stroke may leave the person irresponsive and even in a vegetative state (see page 2). In some cases, depression may trigger the withdrawal. In other cases, losing interest in things and people around, even close family, is a natural part of gradually withdrawing from the world.

Your 'needs' at this difficult time can differ from those of the terminally ill person. You will need to find your own way through. You could, for instance, look back and see how you coped during previous stressful experiences. What helped when, for example, a parent, grandparent or close friend died? What proved a problem? What will you tell your children or grandchildren?

Give yourself permission and time to grieve. Do not expect life to get 'back to normal' too quickly. Profound sadness, a deep sense of loss, sleeplessness, crying, inability to concentrate, tiredness and poor appetite are part of normal grief. They do not mean that you are mentally ill. Tears discharge the tension generated by sadness. According to one estimate, 'resolving' the loss of a loved pet means crying for at least 20 hours. 'Resolving' (you may never overcome) the loss of a spouse, parent, child or close friend requires 200–300 hours of crying.[63]

Occasionally, however, grief goes beyond the 'normal' response to bereavement. You may, for example, develop depression, abuse drugs or alcohol, or feel 'dead' or 'unreal'. You may find you cannot work or take part in your normal activities several weeks after the death, or suffer symptoms of post-traumatic stress disorder (see page 119). If you think your grief is abnormal, speak to your GP or a counsellor: drugs or psychological interventions, such as guided mourning, often help. Talking to your spiritual leader, a counsellor or a member of the palliative care team can also help emotionally and practically. Cruse or the Child Bereavement Trust also offer specific counselling and help for bereaved people.

5

Stroke rehabilitation

Stroke rehabilitation aims to ensure that each survivor reaches his or her maximum physical, functional, psychological and social potential within the limitations caused by any disability.[2] Sometimes, you can make a full or almost complete recovery after a stroke. Louis Pasteur – the great French biologist – developed the rabies vaccine, proved that germs caused infections and invented pasteurization, the process that keeps milk fresh. Pasteur suffered a stroke when he was 47 years old and went on to do some of his most important work.[8]

Lindley comments that the Hollywood star Kirk Douglas 'made a remarkable recovery from a severe stroke'. (You can read more about Douglas's inspiring story at <www.nlm.nih.gov/medline-plus/magazine/issues/summer07/articles/summer07pg8-9.html>. And when the great British dictionary complier Samuel Johnson suffered a stroke on 17 June 1783, he tested his facilities by composing a Latin poem. 'The lines were not very good,' he wrote, 'but I knew them not to be very good.'[7]

Nevertheless, a stroke can cause a wide range of problems (see Table 5.1). This means that rehabilitation is individualized to each person's disability and problems, and draws on the skills of physical, occupational, speech and language therapists as appropriate. This multidisciplinary team works together to help you regain skills, such as speaking or walking, or learn new techniques to compensate for your disability. As a result, this chapter offers an overview of the principles of stroke rehabilitation. You should always follow the specific advice of your stroke rehabilitation team.

However, even with sophisticated imaging equipment, doctors and therapists cannot predict your outcome accurately – even though you and your family are often desperate to know. For example, in the hours and days after a stroke, the brain is swollen and inflamed. Doctors often cannot tell how much of the loss of function is caused by the stroke and how much arises from the

Table 5.1 Examples of problems after a stroke

Difficulty	Per cent of survivors affected
General movement	80
Altered sensation	Up to 80
Arm movement	70
Problems with sight	Up to 66
Long-term inability to use one arm	40
Altered swallowing (dysphagia)	40
Altered speech (aphasia/dysphasia)	33
Spasticity	19–38
Depression	29
Dementia six months after the stroke	20
Pain after the stroke	5–20
Incontinence a year after the stroke	15

Adapted from the Stroke Association

swelling. In general, however, the more rapidly a person begins to improve, the better their long-term prospects.[8] For example, patients who can move their hips within a week after their stroke can usually move around given time, although they might need to use an aid.[2]

Initially, you will probably have at least 45 minutes a day of each therapy that you need over at least five days a week.[5] Rehabilitation should last for as long as you continue to improve. In general, most of the improvement in movement, senses and speech occurs in the first 3–6 months after the stroke. So, you will probably begin rehabilitation as soon as possible.[2] Nevertheless, the UK guidelines note that many survivors find that 'they continue their recovery many months and even years after their stroke', even long after formal rehabilitation ends.[5]

The importance of goals

During rehabilitation, the stroke team will set realistic short- and long-term goals. You and the stroke team will regularly re-evaluate these goals.[2] These goals should be measurable (such as five or ten repetitions of the sit-to-stand exercise, or time spent on an exercise bike), meaningful and relevant to you, and they should help you participate in leisure and family activities. The UK guidelines suggest that the goals should be 'challenging but achievable' and should include short-term goals (days and weeks) and long-term goals (weeks and months). Whenever necessary the goals will include carers. You might want, for example to:

- walk around the shopping centre or go to a match on a Saturday afternoon – walking to the kitchen and the local high street might be a good start;
- speak to your friends and relatives on the phone – you could begin by stating what you want at mealtimes or what you want to wear;
- go on holiday – a short-term goal might be to eat out with friends.[10]

Therapists will pace rehabilitation to match your progress. For example, when you can keep your balance while sitting, rehabilitation might then focus on washing your face and cleaning your teeth. As your recovery continues, rehabilitation will cover tasks such as getting on and off the toilet, dressing and feeding.[7]

Practice makes perfect

The stroke rehabilitation team will develop a programme that helps you meet these goals based on your progress. For example, the therapist may delay walking or other movements if he or she feels that you might reinforce abnormal patterns.[7] So, you should understand *why* the therapist wants you to practise a particular exercise. In some cases, rehabilitation targets a specific problem, such as weak ankles that makes standing and getting around difficult. In other cases, such as washing and dressing, the team may break the activity down into stages.[49] The rehabilitation team then helps survivors translate these skills into everyday activities.[20] At first, however, the exercise may seem a little divorced from your everyday life. You need to understand how it will help in the longer term.

Remaining motivated is easier when you appreciate why you are exercising, especially as progress may seem slow at times. Stroke survivors may also be easily distracted. So try to keep interruptions to a minimum and turn the television off when you exercise or need to focus.

In between your rehabilitation sessions, you can imagine yourself performing the movements and activities. Even exercising in your mind's eye seems to improve physical performance.[5] Indeed, many leading sports people regularly use visualization to improve their performance.

As it's important to know why as well as how to exercise, you and your carer might want to bring a list of questions to discuss with the rehabilitation team.[10] You will often have a lot of information to take on board and, as we have seen, stroke can undermine memory and cognition. Jotting notes during the consultation with a doctor or a therapist and having a list of questions can help. I would suggest talking over the discussions with your relatives or carers once you are at home or back on the ward. This helps consolidate the memory (for you and your carers) and reveals if there is anything you are unsure about. A quick phone call to the stroke team or to a patient group often resolves any uncertainty. You and your carer should know whom to contact if you have any worries.

Get what you are entitled to

Often hospitals face considerable pressure to discharge people quickly. Most people want to come home as soon as possible. However, families and stroke survivors may overestimate how well they can cope, especially as support from community health and social services may be limited. You should receive clear advice about your rights, benefits and support.[64] If you do not, ask. A social worker can help you and your carer access the benefits, transport, voluntary services and so on that help rehabilitation.

Cognitive impairment

Up to 60 per cent of stroke survivors show some impairment in cognition, which is essentially the ability to think, remember and plan.[12] Indeed, while lacunar strokes (see page 12) affect only a relatively small area of brain, cognitive problems are still common.

When researchers looked at 24 studies, they found that 30 per cent of people are cognitively impaired in the four years after a lacunar stroke. This is similar to the rate (23 per cent) among those who survived a non-lacunar stroke, despite non-lacunar strokes tending to affect a larger area of the brain and, typically, being more severe. However, many lacunar strokes arise from age-related changes in the small blood vessels supplying the brain. Some of the same changes can cause dementia by reducing blood flow to the brain (so-called vascular dementia). This overlap may account for the similar rate of cognitive impairment in people who survive lacunar and non-lacunar strokes.[65] Indeed, stroke itself can double the likelihood of dementia[27] and is now the second most common cause of dementia, after Alzheimer's disease.[7]

Give your memory a boost

You can give your memory a helping hand in several ways, including:[10]

- trying memory aids, such as making lists or using a diary, for things and events that you need to remember;
- fixing a routine – such as meal times, when you have a take-away or ask a relative or friend to call;
- breaking up tasks – such as getting dressed, making lunch or doing laundry – into a series of steps using a list or pictures;
- sticking notes or pictures on important cupboards and drawers, such as where you keep foods, drinks and cutlery;
- practising your mental skills by craftwork and board games. Craftwork can also help your manual dexterity – as always, it is best to start with simple tasks and move on to more complicated activities as you improve.

These are only a few examples. A clinical psychologist can identify your particular pattern of cognitive problems and find tailored ways to overcome issues such as poor memory, poor concentration and poor attention as well as difficulties with orientation around the day and time.

Don't mistake apraxia for being awkward

Some strokes damage the part of the brain that allows people to translate ideas into actions – a problem called apraxia. As a result, people with apraxia cannot voluntarily perform skilled movements despite being physically strong enough and retaining adequate sensation.[5,10]

For example, a person with apraxia may not be able to make a cup of tea or even use a spoon at the right time.[5] In some cases, people with apraxia can perform the movement – such as putting a jumper on – when they do not think about it, but not when asked. They may get out of a chair when asked to come into the kitchen, but not when asked to stand up. It's important not to mistake apraxia for stubbornness or 'manipulative behaviour'.[10]

Language problems

We have all had that irritating feeling of a word being right on the tip of our tongue. Imagine experiencing that all the time. That's the problem experienced by many stroke survivors with dysphasia – also called aphasia. Originally, 'aphasia' meant a total loss of the ability to use and understand written or spoken words. Dysphasia referred to a less severe problem. Today, the two terms are used interchangeably.[3]

For example, a survivor may know what he or she wants to say but just not be able to find the right words – this is 'expressive dysphasia'. Some survivors cannot even call for help if they get into difficulty. Other people with expressive dysphasia can understand speech and speak reasonably well. However, they may have problems naming objects or people.[7]

Other stroke survivors experience problems understanding what other people say – so-called 'receptive dysphasia'. You can get an idea of what this is like by thinking back to when you were on holiday or watching a foreign film and heard people speaking in a language you do not understand. You knew they were talking to each other. At best, you recognize a few words. In some cases, people who lose their ability to understand language speak without hesitation, but use words incorrectly, speak gibberish or 'don't say anything', or make up words. This 'fluent dysphasia' is often associated with severe problems in understanding.[3,7]

Unfortunately, dysphasia is common. Around a third of survivors develop dysphasia soon after their stroke.[5] About 12 per cent still show dysphasia 6 months later.[2] Dysphasia makes things harder for the person as they rebuild their relationships, occupation and leisure activities. Not surprisingly, many survivors and their carers find speech problems among the most difficult disabilities to cope with. Indeed, stroke survivors with speech loss are the most likely to develop depression (see page 43).

In other cases, communication problems arise when a stroke damages the muscles in the face. This means that the stroke survivor may have problems forming words because of slow, weak, imprecise and uncoordinated muscle movements – a problem called dysarthria. For example, try saying 'b', 'f', 'm', 'p', 'v' or 'w' without moving your lips. You cannot. If a stroke damages the person's ability to move the lips, he or she may have problems saying 'bottle' (which is why bad ventriloquists say 'gottle of geer'), 'minute', 'family' and so on.[66] Many people with dysarthria also experience swallowing problems.

Dysphonia arises when the stroke affects muscles in the voice box. The survivor can have problems forming words or controlling the volume of their voice.

A speech and language therapist will assess and manage the particular problem. For example, the therapist may be able to teach the survivor to use gestures, word-and-picture cards, symbols, and computers and smart phone apps to aid communication.[10]

Communication aid

If you are speaking to a stroke survivor:[3,10]

- Do not raise your voice unless you know that their hearing is poor. If you find you have to raise your voice a lot, it might be worth checking whether the survivor needs a hearing aid or if the current device is working properly.
- If you (or the stroke survivor) wears dentures, you should make sure they still fit properly. This makes speaking easier.
- Do not speak to the survivor as if you are talking to are a child. Just because a person cannot speak, that does not mean that he or she does not understand. However, it is worth gently checking that the stroke survivor understands what the carer is saying and vice versa.
- Speak slowly. You may sometimes find that you need to repeat what you say. However, try to rephrase things, rather than just say the same thing over and over.
- Try to establish eye contact. The survivor can watch your face and lips, which helps understanding.

- Listen to the survivor, but do not pretend to understand what he or she is saying. This just creates confusion. You could ask the survivor to point or use gestures.
- Resist the temptation to speak for the survivor when you are with family, friends or on a day out.
- Reduce distractions, such as the television or radio, when you are trying to communicate.

With practice and patience, even people with relatively severe problems can often learn to communicate again.

Sensory changes

Up to 80 per cent of stroke survivors report loss or alterations in their senses, including reduced touch, unpleasant feelings of hot, cold or tingling (pins and needles), and pain. People with more extensive motor problems tend to show more severe sensory loss.[5] In other words, the two complications seem to be related.

Therapists typically use two approaches to 're-train' senses. Passive re-training uses electrical stimulation to improve function and reduce pain. Active re-training repeatedly exposures the survivor to different stimuli, including texture, temperature, joint position or shape.[5]

Difficulty swallowing

During the first few weeks and months after a stroke, you do not need to worry unduly about eating a healthy diet. Ensuring you get enough calories and nutrients often poses enough of a challenge. Indeed, up to 30 per cent of survivors have a poor diet and show malnutrition and dehydration after a stroke.[5] So, if you cannot take adequate amounts of food and water by mouth within 24 hours of reaching hospital, the staff may insert a nasogastric tube, which runs from your nose into your stomach.[3]

Dysphagia (difficulty swallowing), limited arm movement, poor dental hygiene, depression, anxiety, fatigue and unfamiliar foods can all contribute to poor nutrition after a stroke.[5] For example, depending on the method used to assess swallowing, between 37 and 78 per cent of stroke survivors develop dysphagia.[67]

So, when a person reaches hospital with a suspected stroke, a doctor or nurse will assess the person's ability to swallow[20] by, for example, asking the person to drink a glass of water to see if he or she coughs or chokes. A speech and language therapist or another experienced healthcare professional will assess swallowing ability in detail once the person is out of immediate danger. Furthermore, several medicines can cause a dry mouth because of lack of saliva (xerostomia),[68] which makes swallowing difficult.

Tragically, dysphagia after a stroke is not diagnosed in 80 per cent of survivors with swallowing problems and they do not receive any specific treatment.[67] So, carers and stroke survivors should watch for signs that might indicate dysphagia, such as:

- difficulty controlling food in the mouth;
- problems swallowing;
- coughing or choking;
- gurgling or a wet voice after swallowing;
- nasal regurgitation;
- feeling that the food 'becomes stuck' or is 'held up'.

Sometimes the signs are less obvious or the person may just push the plate away. However, dysphagia is not the only cause of appetite loss in stroke survivors. If you suspect that you or the person you care for has swallowing problems ask your GP for a referral to a speech and language therapist or a dietician experienced in assessing swallowing problems.

The stages of swallowing

A healthy person swallows about 600 times a day, usually when eating or drinking, but also approximately 50 times while asleep.[69] Chewing forms a bolus of food. The tongue moves the bolus towards the back of the mouth. This is the 'pre-swallow' phase. Swallowing comprises three stages – oral, pharyngeal and oesophageal – during which co-ordinated movements transport the bolus through the pharynx, down the oesophagus and into the stomach.[69] A stroke that affects any one of these stages can lead to swallowing problems.

Aspiration pneumonia

In about half of people with dysphagia, swallowing problems improve during the week after the stroke. Dysphagia persists in the remainder, who are vulnerable to distressing complications.[67] For example, up to 25 per cent of people with post-stroke dysphagia develop malnutrition, dehydration or both, and up to 20 per cent of stroke survivors experience aspiration pneumonia,[67] which is a major cause of death during the year after the stroke. Aspiration – breathing food, saliva, liquids or vomit into the lungs – encourages the growth of bacteria, leading to pneumonia (infection of the lungs)).[67]

Infections are relatively common after a stroke. Up to 65 per cent of stroke survivors develop a related infection, including urinary tract infections (about 23 per cent of survivors; page 83) and chest infections (about 22 per cent). Aspiration pneumonia causes many of these chest infections. About half of survivors who have dysphagia develop aspiration, for example. More than a third of these develop aspiration pneumonia.[3]

Helping food go down

If you continue to have problems, a dietician can work out a meal plan to provide food that is easy to swallow. Minced, mashed and pureed food can compensate for fatigue, chewing and swallowing problems. You can purchase 'ready meals' specifically prepared for people with swallowing problems.

Safely swallowing water, tea and other thin liquids requires particularly fine co-ordination of muscles and nerves.[70] So, your dietician or stroke team may suggest adding thickeners to water, juice and other thin drinks. Some people find carbonation of fluids or changing the temperature helps. Following the safe swallowing tips (see Table 5.2), whether you feed yourself or someone helps, also makes feeding easier and safer.

An occupational therapist will help you find the best position in which to eat. Tucking your chin in may help, for example. In addition, speech and language therapists can teach alternative swallowing manoeuvres and suggest exercises to improve swallowing tailored to your needs and circumstances (such as the swallowing stage affected). At first, for example, you may have swallowing therapy at least three times a week. Treatment is likely to continue for as long as you continue to improve.

Table 5.2   Safe swallowing tips

Do not mix food and drink in the same mouthful
Do not talk while you are eating
Keep each mouthful small: this may mean you only eat or drink a teaspoon's worth at a time
Sit upright for half an hour after each meal
Swallow each mouthful before eating or drinking any more
Take your time; mealtimes should be relaxed and quiet
Try eating smaller meals more frequently, rather than three larger meals a day

Adapted from the Stroke Association

Movement problems

Between 70 and 88 per cent of people who experience an ischaemic stroke develop motor (movement) problems.[2] However, the type and severity of movement disorder depends on the area of the brain damaged by the stroke. So, strokes can cause a variety of movement problems including:

- hemiplegia – weaknesses on one side of the body; according to the UK stroke guidelines, weakness on one side of the body 'is probably the single most disabling factor, certainly in terms of limiting mobility';[5]
- hemiballism – vigorous, irregular and marked limb movements on one side of the body;[71]
- chorea – brief, arrhythmic, non-repetitive movements that appear to move from muscle to muscle;[71]
- dystonia – involuntary sustained twisting, repetitive movements or abnormal postures; younger people – those aged less than 25 years – seem to be especially prone to dystonia;[71]
- spasticity – abnormal increase in muscle tone (see page 79).

These problems do not always emerge soon after the stroke. Hemiballism, for example, typically develops around the time of the stroke. However, dystonia tends to emerge, on average, 9.5 months after the stroke, but it can emerge up to three years later. People with hemiplegia often develop dystonia once their muscle strength begins to recover. Although dystonia often stabilizes, this movement disorder rarely totally resolves.[71]

Survivors should, in general, begin to get back on their feet and move within 24 hours of the stroke.[5] Immobility, even for a short time, can lead to a variety of problems, including muscle wastage, reduced movement, slower wound healing, problems urinating and pressure sores (pressure ulcers).[49] For example, about 21 per cent of stroke survivors develop pressure sores while in hospital, compared with between 4 per cent and 10 per cent of those with other conditions.[3] As we have seen (see page 51), the greater likelihood of early activity is one reason why outcomes in specialist stroke units are especially good.

Treating movement disorders

Ninety per cent of movement disorders that emerge soon after the stroke resolve within 6 months. Nevertheless, many people need help getting around, at least in the short term. The rehabilitation team will train carers in, for example, safely transferring the survivor – such as getting out of bed or getting up from a chair – and make sure the carer and survivor can use assistance devices, including those needed to get around and for feeding.[2]

Arming yourself against movement problems

About 70 per cent of patients experience altered arm function after a stroke. Approximately 40 per cent show persistent disability in their arms. Therapy – such as high-intensity, repetitive and task-specific training – can help.[5] Unfortunately, the hand's fine movements often recover very slowly and often do not reach the dexterity the survivor had before the stroke.[8]

To maximize the chances of recovery a therapist may give you a mitt that you wear over your good hand. This forces you to use the hand affected by your stroke. Other approaches include:

- stimulating the affected muscles with a mild electrical current;[2]
- using certain drugs; for example, haloperidol – often used to treat schizophrenia – was shown to resolve symptoms in 56 per cent of patients with hemiballism in between three and 15 days;[71]
- using splints and other externally applied devices (orthoses) to improve function and movement, or reduce pain.

Splints

A splint or orthoses can increase your range of movement if, for example, your muscles and tendons permanently shorten. This problem (called a contracture) can cause abnormal and often painful postures.[49] An orthoses can help correct an abnormal shape of a limb affected by a contracture. Ankle–foot orthoses or strapping help maintain you stability as you stand and move around.[49] Hand and wrist splints can also:

- help you grip;
- allow you or your carer to reach your palm to make sure it is clean; and
- stop your fingernails from digging into your palm.

You or your family should know how and when to remove the splint or orthosis and watch for redness and other signs of skin damage. The skin can become broken and develop into an open sore that is often very hard to heal. You should speak to the rehabilitation team or your GP if you are concerned.

Robotic arms

Computer-controlled automated devices that can move a limb – essentially robots – potentially respond as the person's needs change. The automated arms can help rehabilitation, such as helping the survivor to relearn grasping skills[72] or offering additional support.

At the start of 2013, more than 120 rehabilitation devices were available for arm disability alone, ranging from simple braces to exoskeletons.[72] Currently, UK guidelines suggest using robot-assisted movement in combination with conventional therapy to reduce arm impairment.[5] Numerous clinical studies are assessing robotic and related technology, and their use is likely to grow over the next few years.

Falls

About 40 per cent of stroke survivors fall at least once during their rehabilitation.[2] About a fifth of these falls result in injury.[2] As a result, survivors are about seven times more likely to break a bone in the year after the stroke compared to the general population.[26] Fortunately, the risk decreases after the first year.[26]

Certain stroke survivors seem especially likely to fall, including those with hemi-neglect (see page 80) or movement problems. Almost four out of every five survivors who depend on other people for the activities of daily living fall in the first six months at home.[3]

Some anticoagulants (see page 52) and a lack of weight-bearing by a disabled limb seem to weaken the bones,[26] which increases the risk of a fracture if you are unfortunate enough to fall. Carers need to know how to prevent falls, how to help someone up and how to make appropriate adaptations around the home.

Spasticity

A balance of nerve signals controls each muscle. One set of signals tells your muscles to contact. Another tells the muscles to relax. A stroke can disrupt this balance. For example, if a stroke damages signals telling the muscles to contract, your limbs may be limp, flaccid and floppy. If a stroke damages the signals telling the muscles to relax, you may develop stiffness and involuntary muscle spasms, a problem called spasticity.[73]

In many cases, muscles stay contracted for long periods, remaining stiff and tight. The contraction can pull joints into abnormal positions or prevent the normal range of motion. Other stroke survivors develop rapid muscle contractions (clonus), exaggerated reflexes, muscle spasms, scissoring (involuntary crossing of the legs) and 'locked' joints. Untreated, muscles affected by spasticity can develop contracture and can limit the success of rehabilitation.[73]

A common problem

One study examined 211 patients six months after their first ischaemic stroke: almost 43 per cent developed spasticity. About 16 per cent showed severe spasticity, especially in the arms rather than the legs.[11] Another study found that spasticity was especially common in the elbow (79 per cent of patients with the problem), wrist (66 per cent) and ankle (66 per cent).[73]

Treating spasticity usually includes physical therapy and, in some cases, surgery and drugs that relax muscle and botulium toxin (see page 54). Botulium toxin relaxes muscle and improves tone. For example, by allowing the ankle or arm to function more normally, the person's mobility can improve. Some people find that ice massage and heat packs help alleviate spasticity.[10]

Vision

Half of all nerves reaching the brain begin in the eyes.[74] So, not surprisingly, stroke survivors may experience problems with sight – including double vision, blurred vision, poor depth perception and nystagmus (continuous, uncontrolled eye movement).

Doctors call loss of the visual field (how much you can see at any time) on one side of the body hemianopia. Usually, you lose the same area of vision in both eyes – called homonymous hemianopia. Stroke accounts for about 70 per cent of cases of homonymous hemianopia. Tumours, haemorrhages in the eye and other problems cause the remainder.[74]

Hemi-neglect

Patients may differ in their levels of awareness between the two sides of the body (hemi-neglect). Doctors can test for hemi-neglect by asking the survivor to cross out all the lines on a page, draw a clock, copy a figure or mark the exact centre of a line.[2] However, hemi-neglect does not necessarily arise from damage to the brain's visual areas. The areas in the brain that receive signals from the eye may not be able to process even accurate information. While the person 'sees' the side they do not 'know' that they see it.

About 10 per cent of people with post-stroke visual disturbances recover completely. Another 50 per cent recover partially. Most of the recovery takes place in the first 48 hours after a stroke and further improvement without help (see below) after 3 months is very unlikely.[74]

Hemianopia can lead to difficulty balancing or with co-ordination. In some cases, the person may have problems recognizing things or people, which can be distressing for family and friends. Furthermore, left hemianopia or hemi-neglect can pose a particular problem when, for example, reading. The left parts of a word contain more information needed than the right (at least in English). So, people with left-sided hemianopia or hemi-neglect tend to make more mistakes when reading by misidentifying the initial part of a word.[74]

Try staring at this letter: **A**. You probably don't realize that your eyes were not still even when you stared at the letter. Whether still, reading or glancing around, your eyes make rapid movements called saccades that scan the area. Strokes can reduce the number of saccades and, therefore, you take longer to evaluate a scene visually. This makes navigating around more difficult[10] and can contribute to hemianopia or hemi-neglect.

Help for hemianopia and hemi-neglect

Your rehabilitation team can offer a lot of help for people with hemianopia or hemi-neglect. For example:

- Physiotherapists and occupational therapists can help you compensate for areas of blindness or neglect. For example, 'vision exploration training' can help survivors develop strategies to search a visual field.[74] Even just moving the head from side-to-side allows people to scan areas on the 'damaged' side.[10]
- A clinical psychologist can help you find new ways to process information – such as recognizing things or people.
- An ophthalmologist or optician can offer visual aids. For example, spectacles that include a prism can shift objects from, for instance, the left towards the right to compensate for hemi-neglect.[2] This make help you avoid obstacles (thereby, reducing the risk of a fall – see page 78) and make it easier to find things.[74] Survivors may also have eye problems unrelated to the stroke – such as cataracts, glaucoma and suboptimal glasses – which makes matters worse. So, always get your eyes tested.
- You can request large print books and audio books: try your local library, bookshop or on-line retailer.
- Brightly coloured lines or running a highlighter along the edge of the page can draw attention to the neglected side.
- If people cannot perceive items on one side, place the most important items on the other side. For example, if they have left-sided hemi-neglect try placing their clothes on the right side of drawers and cupboards.

Incontinence and urinary problems

Between 32 and 79 per cent of survivors experience urinary incontinence at least for a short time after their stroke.[2,3] Some do not get to the toilet in time. Some make it in time, but feel they have a desperate need to pass urine (so-called urgency) or a need to pass urine often (frequency). In addition, between 30 and 56 per cent of stroke survivors have faecal incontinence.[26]

In most people, bladder and bowel control improves over time.[26] Nevertheless, about 20 per cent of survivors have urinary incontinence 6 months after their stroke.[3] Some people who cannot pass water properly need a catheter inserted into their bladder. Because a catheter increases the risk of infections and other complications, doctors will leave this in for the shortest time possible.

Incontinence after a stroke has several causes including:[26]

- damage to the nerves controlling the bladder and bowel;
- changes in diet;
- being bedbound;
- difficulty communicating to carers that they need to use the toilet;
- mobility problems that mean they cannot get to the toilet in time;
- brain damage that means the person is less aware that they need to go to the toilet;
- certain medicines.

Again, the expert rehabilitation team can make a big difference. For example:

- A specialist nurse, called a continence adviser, can help re-train the bladder using pelvic floor exercises. These exercises strengthen muscles around the bladder and urethra allowing you to hold on to the urine until you reach the toilet. The continence adviser can also suggest aids, such as pads and bed covers.
- Physiotherapists can improve your mobility and so help you use the toilet or commode.
- Occupational therapists may be able to suggest adaptations that make using the toilet easier, such as making the seat higher.
- Doctors can prescribe drugs that help with some types of urinary incontinence.

• Reducing the amount of caffeine you drink may also help.[3] Try plain water, fruit juices and herbal teas instead.

Watch for urinary tract infections

About a quarter of stroke survivors develop a urinary tract infection (UTI).[3] However, you are three to four times more likely to develop a UTI if you need a catheter compared to other stroke survivors.[3] But everyone – whether or not they use a catheter – should see their GP if they develop any of the following:[10]

• urinary incontinence or retention (you cannot urinate);
• you urinate much more or less often than usual;
• urination hurts or your lower back hurts;
• change in the colour of your urine – such as being bloody or brown;
• urine that smells;
• urine that seems to have a different consistency from usual or that contains a sediment;
• other signs of an infection, such as chills or a fever.

Pain

Many people endure considerable pain after a stroke, although communication and cognitive difficulties can make the extent of the discomfort difficult for doctors to ascertain. For example, a part of the brain called the thalamus processes pain signals received from the rest of the body. Strokes affecting the thalamus and other areas that process pain cause 'central pain', a problem that develops in between 2 and 8 per cent of survivors.

Central pain can emerge soon after a stroke or, more commonly, several weeks or months later. Often central pain seems to develop in a weakened part of a body, such as an arm or leg. Commonly, the damage to the pain processing areas exaggerates the effect of stimulation: a light touch evokes painful sensations that may feel like a toothache or like a searing, burning, itching or stretching pain.[7] Conventional painkillers – even potent analgesics such as morphine – are often ineffective against this sort of pain. However, pregabalin and gabapentin (also used to treat epilepsy) usually alleviate the discomfort.[5]

Problems with muscles and joints (for example, arising from spasticity or changes in gait) and depression can trigger or exacerbate pain. Up to 80 per cent of stroke survivors develop shoulder pain, for instance, which can disturb sleep, yet may dissipate only after rest. Up to 25 per cent develop a condition called shoulder-hand syndrome: in addition to marked shoulder pain, the hand becomes painful, swollen and discoloured. Shoulder-hand syndrome typically develops about 1 or 2 months after the stroke.[2]

Of course, other problems (such as arthritis) can cause pain.[5] So, try to communicate the extent and site of your pain. If you are a carer ask about pain. Don't wait to be told.

Acupuncture

Acupuncture is not widely available as part of NHS rehabilitation, despite a growing number of studies suggesting it might help some stroke survivors. Acupuncture is, for example, a well-established pain treatment[75] and may alleviate specific stroke symptoms.

One study looked at 20,923 cases of paralysis caused by stroke that were treated with acupuncture of the scalp. Practitioners inserted the needles into a part of the scalp that acupuncturists call the 'motor area'. Almost 37 per cent of stroke people were 'cured', another 34 per cent showed marked improvements and 25 per cent showed some improvement. Another study looked at 1,800 people treated with scalp acupuncture for stroke-related paralysis: almost 26 per cent recovered fully, 53 per cent markedly improved and 16 per cent somewhat improved. Only 5 per cent failed to show a benefit. Practitioners also claim that most people show at least some improvement after scalp acupuncture for swallowing problems.[76] Unfortunately, we do not know how many people in these studies would have recovered anyway. But acupuncture could be worth a try.

Nevertheless, despite intensive research, it is not yet clear why acupuncture works. A paper in the prestigious *Archives of Internal Medicine* considered 31 studies – which included almost 18,000 patients – and reported that acupuncture roughly halved the intensity of chronic pain caused by back, neck and shoulder problems, osteoarthritis and headache. Yet, the paper points out, 'there is no accepted mechanism by which [acupuncture] could have persisting effects on chronic pain'.[75] Nevertheless, these promising results suggest that scalp acupuncture might be worth considering in addition to your conventional rehabilitation, after mentioning it to your rehabilitation team. Contact the British Medical Acupuncture Society or the British Acupuncture Council.

Headaches

Between 34 and 60 per cent of people experience headaches following haemorrhagic strokes and between 25 and 44 per cent after TIAs. Headaches are less common after ischaemic strokes, affecting between 4 and 31 per cent of people. The cause of headaches in stroke is unclear,[77] although painkillers or other drugs can often help.

Seizures and epilepsy

About 5–10 per cent of people develop seizure disorders (epilepsy) linked to a stroke.[2,10] Indeed, strokes are the most common reason why seizures emerge for the first time in elderly people.[7] Seizures arise from bouts of uncontrolled electrical activity in the brain. This causes tingling and twitching in, for example, an arm or a leg. The classic seizures – a 'grand mal' or tonic–clonic seizure, in which the person loses consciousness and twitches uncontrollably on the ground – are rare after a stroke unless the person previously had epilepsy.[10]

A seizure is one of the first symptoms of about one in 50 strokes. Unfortunately, seizures can complicate diagnosis. A brain tumour, withdrawal from alcohol and drugs, an abscess in the brain and a variety of other conditions can also cause seizures. In addition, some seizure disorders can mimic strokes.[7] In a few cases, you may need to take anticonvulsants to control the seizures after a stroke.

6

Lifestyle changes to prevent another stroke

Humans did not evolve to chomp on 'junk food' high in sugar and fat, and sparse in nutrients. We evolved to eat a diet rich in fruit and vegetables, and low in animal fats. The Kitava people of Papua New Guinea, for example, follow a traditional subsistence diet and lifestyle. In the early 1990s, researchers could not find a single Kitavan who had suffered a stroke. Indeed, none of the Kitavans could recall anyone dying with symptoms that could indicate a stroke.[7]

Closer to home, the Mediterranean diet:

- is rich in olive oil and canola (rapeseed) oil;
- is low in cholesterol and saturated (animal) fat;
- contains large amounts of whole grains, fruit, vegetables, lentils, beans and nuts; and
- uses fish rather than red meat as a source of protein.

As we shall see, recent studies underscore the importance of eating sufficient protein to help prevent stroke (see page 95). Nevertheless, the traditional Mediterranean diet contains less animal protein than the typical 'Western' diet and limits red meat to less than once a week. Several studies suggest that this traditional Mediterranean diet protects against stroke in particular and cardiovascular disease more generally.[78]

However, food is more than just a source of energy and nutrients: it has a central role in our culture and society. Animals consume almost anything that is available and that their experience and senses deem edible. Human culture and society determine what food is acceptable, and when. Guinea pigs, whales, horse and dog are acceptable foods in certain cultures but usually inspire revulsion in the English-speaking world. And how often do you eat plum pudding and brandy butter or Brussels sprouts unless it's Christmas? Cooking – and food preparation generally – transforms nature into culture. There's no good reason to boil cabbage, for example, and certain styles of cooking and food preparation symbolize social status.[79] Having tried *nouvelle cuisine* in London restaurants, the fact that I would much rather eat fish and chips in Hunstanton, Aldeburgh or Whitley Bay probably says more about me than the relative merits of these two culinary traditions.

Despite food's social importance, stroke survivors who develop dysphagia may insist on eating alone, partly because of embarrassment about their disability. This means that they lose the pleasure associated with the social and recreational benefits of eating – and not just on birthdays, anniversaries and Christmas. Regularly eating together helps forge bonds between families and partners.

A nutritious diet is important to help you recover after a stroke. So, during the first few weeks and months after a stroke, your dietician will suggest the most appropriate diet to aid your recovery – and that may be higher in calories, for example, than the guidelines for healthy eating suggest. Nevertheless, once you have recovered from your stroke or TIA, healthy eating, quitting smoking and controlling alcohol consumption can help prevent another or your first stroke, even if your other risk factors mean that you are at high risk.

Cooking safely after a stoke

Cooking can be difficult and dangerous after a stroke. For example, memory problems may mean that stroke survivors wander off leaving the cooking. Survivors may spill hot food or liquids: weakness or poor dexterity can make moving pots, plates and pans difficult. Sliding is safer than lifting. A splatter screen can reduce the risk. If you use a wheelchair, a mirror can help you see into the pans. A hotplate, microwave and toaster oven may be safer than a conventional cooker.[10] Your occupational therapist should be able to suggest changes that make cooking easier and safer given your particular problems.

Changing your diet, even if it's good for you, can seem daunting. However, many people find that it takes only a month or so of eating – or not eating – a food for the change to become a habit. Some people (myself among them) who switch to skimmed milk from full-fat milk soon find that they dislike the taste of full-fat milk. Similarly, many people soon lose their sweet tooth or their taste for salt – and salt is one of the most important dietary causes of stroke.

Reducing salt

High-salt diets are a leading cause of hypertension and, therefore, stroke. Each extra 5 grams of salt you eat each day increases stroke risk by 23 per cent. Between 2003 and 2011 salt intake in England decreased by 1.4 grams a day, a 15 per cent reduction. Nevertheless, during 2011, average salt intake (8.1 grams a day) was still 35 per cent higher than recommended (6 grams a day). Indeed, 80 per cent of men and 58 per cent women consumed more that the recommended level of salt.[1] But you should follow your doctor's advice: some people (for example, those with liver disease, heart failure or hypertension) need to eat even less than this.

You soon know that crisps and peanuts are salty. However, many foods contain 'hidden salt': your taste buds will not set alarm bells ringing. For example, manufacturers add surprisingly large amounts of salt to some soups, bread, biscuits, processed meat (including ham and salami), cheese, stock cubes and even ice cream.[5,7] Indeed, salt added to processed foods accounts for approximately 80 per cent of our total salt intake.[1] So:[10]

- read the label and try to stick to low-salt foods;
- avoid foods – such as smoked meat and fish – that are high in salt;
- add as little salt as you can during baking and cooking;
- banish the salt cellar from the table;
- ask restaurants and take-aways for 'no salt';
- check levels of added salt and fat for 'self-basting' poultry;
- look for low-salt ketchup, pickles, mustard, yeast extract, stock cubes and so on;
- avoid foods that include a chemical name that includes sodium, such as disodium phosphate, monosodium glutamate or sodium nitrate.

The British Dietetic Association advises choosing meals and sandwiches with less than 0.5 grams of sodium (1.25 grams of salt) per

Table 6.1   Salt levels in food

Level of salt	Salt content	Sodium content
High	More than 1.5 grams per 100 grams of food	More than 0.6 grams per 100 grams of food
Medium	0.3–1.5 grams per 100 grams of food	0.1–0.6 grams per 100 grams of food
Low	0.3 grams or less per 100 grams of food	0.1 grams or less per 100 grams of food

Adapted from the British Dietetic Association

meal. Choose individual foods – such as soups and sauces – with less than 0.3 grams of sodium (0.75 grams of salt) per serving. Some labels list sodium, rather than salt. To convert sodium to salt, multiply by 2.5. So, 0.4 grams of sodium is 1 gram of salt. You can convert salt to sodium by dividing by 2.5 (see Table 6.1).

Usually, reducing salt over a month or so means that you will not notice the change in taste. However, cutting salt is easier said than done for some survivors. As we have seen, stroke can cause profound deficits in the senses, including smell and taste. So, some survivors begin adding unhealthy amounts of salt to their food to improve the taste. In one case, a woman added up to 110 grams of salt a day to her food to stop it tasting bland.[80]

However, learning how to use herbs and spices can help reduce salt consumption, according to a study presented at a meeting run by the American Heart Association during 2014. In the first phase of the study, 55 volunteers ate a low-sodium diet supplied by the researchers for four weeks. Sodium intake decreased from, on average, 3.5 to 1.7 grams a day.

About half the people received lessons showing them how to use herbs and spices in recipes and how to make changes that ensure they follow a low-sodium diet permanently. For example, they learnt how to change traditional recipes to remove salt and include herbs and spices. The researchers encouraged participants to try different herbs and spices. Sodium intake increased in both groups when they stopped using the low-salt diet supplied by the researchers. However, those who received the additional help consumed, on average, about 1 gram of sodium less than those that didn't. If your food seems bland, you could, for example, attend a culinary evening class or work through a range of cookbooks to increase the amount and variety of spices and herbs you use.

Fruit and vegetables

Eating sufficient fruit and vegetables is the bedrock of a healthy diet and can cut the likelihood of stroke (see Table 6.2). For example, researchers looked at 20 studies involving 760,629 people. Those who ate the most fruit and vegetables were 21 per cent less likely to have an ischaemic stroke and 22 per cent less likely to have a haemorrhagic stroke than those who ate the least. Fruit seemed to have a greater effect (23 per cent) than vegetables (14 per cent). Considered separately, the highest intakes of citrus fruits (28 per cent), apples or pears (12 per cent) and leafy vegetables (12 per cent) significantly reduced stroke risk.[81]

Table 6.2   Effect of fruit and vegetables on stroke risk

Diet	Reduction in stroke risk
200 grams *more* fruit a day	32 per cent
200 grams *more* vegetables a day	11 per cent
50 grams of fruits a day	10 per cent
400 grams of fruits a day	55 per cent
50 grams of vegetables a day	3 per cent
400 grams of vegetables a day	20 per cent

Adapted from Hu et al.[81]

Table 6.3   Examples of a portion of fruit and vegetables

One medium-sized fruit (banana, apple, pear, orange)
One slice of a large fruit (melon, pineapple, mango)
Two smaller fruits (plums, satsumas, apricots, peaches)
A dessert bowl full of salad
Three heaped tablespoons of vegetables
Three heaped tablespoons of pulses (chickpeas, lentils, beans)
Two to three tablespoons ('a handful') of grapes or berries
One tablespoon of dried fruit
One glass (150 millilitres) of unsweetened fruit or vegetable juice or smoothie (two or more glasses of juice a day still counts as one portion)

In 2011, the average consumption of fruit and vegetables in the UK was 3.8 portions a day[1] – about 300 grams. This is far short of the dieticians' general recommendation that we eat five portions of fruit and vegetables a day. (A portion weighs about 80 grams.) However, some researchers now believe we should eat at least seven portions of fruit and vegetables a day[82] – almost twice the average intake. Table 6.3 gives some examples of a portion of fruit or vegetables.

Cooking can leach nutrients from fruit and vegetables. So, either eat fruit raw or cook vegetables using a small amount of unsalted water for the shortest time you can. Steaming and stir-frying also preserves nutrients, and scrub rather than peel potatoes, carrots and so on: the skin often contains valuable nutrients.

Why fruit and vegetables reduce stroke risk

Fruit and vegetables are rich in vitamins, minerals and other nutrients, as well as fibre, which seems to account for their protective effects. Increasing dietary potassium consumption – for example, by eating more fruit and vegetables, or using potassium salt substitutes – reduces blood pressure and seems to ameliorate other harmful changes in the vessels and blood that predispose to stroke and cardiovascular disease more widely.[83]

Indeed, overwhelming evidence now shows that a diet rich in fruit and vegetables reduces blood pressure, a leading cause of stroke. For example, researchers combined 39 studies looking at the effect of a vegetarian diet on blood pressure. In this analysis, 'vegetarian' meant that the person did not eat, or only rarely ate, meat from cattle, pigs, sheep and other land animals. Some vegetarian diets in the analysis included dairy products, eggs and fish. On average, vegetarian diets reduced systolic blood pressure by between 4.8 and 6.9 mmHg and diastolic blood pressure by between 2.2 and 4.7 mmHg compared to the normal mixed diet.[84]

Boost your fibre intake

Bowel changes are common among stroke survivors. For instance, up to 60 per cent of stroke survivors develop constipation at some time during their recovery.[3] Some painkillers (especially opioids) can also cause constipation. However, a high-fibre diet can help tackle constipation.

A diet rich in fruit and vegetables is high in fibre (roughage), the part of plants that humans cannot digest, such as the outer layers of sweet corn, beans, wheat and corn. There are two main types of fibre:

- Insoluble fibre remains largely intact as it moves through your digestive system. Insoluble fibre eases defaecation.
- Soluble fibre dissolves in water in the gut, forming a gel that soaks up fats. So, you absorb less fat from a meal, lowering your blood cholesterol levels. Soluble fibre also releases sugar slowly, which staves off hunger pangs and helps you lose weight.

Dieticians recommend that healthy adults eat at least 18 grams of fibre a day. Currently, the average UK adult eats about 14 grams of fibre a day. So, boost your consumption of oats and oat bran, fruit and vegetables, nuts and seeds, pulses (such as peas, soya, lentils and chickpeas) and so on.

Whole grains

Whole grains are an especially rich source of fibre. Grains – the seeds of cereals, such as wheat, rye, barley, oats and rice – have three areas:

- Bran, the outer layer, is rich in fibre and packed with nutrients. Bran covers the 'germ' and endosperm.
- The germ develops into a new plant and is rich in nutrients. Wheat germ, for example, contains high levels of vitamin E, folate (folic acid), zinc, magnesium and other vitamins and minerals.
- The central area (endosperm) is high in starch and provides the energy the germ needs to develop into a new plant.

Many food manufacturers refine grain by stripping off the bran and germ, and keeping the white endosperm. However, refining removes most of the nutrients: whole grains contain up to 75 per cent more nutrients than refined cereals, the British Dietetic Association points out.

Regularly eating whole grains as part of a low-fat diet and a healthy lifestyle cuts the risk of heart disease by up to 30 per cent. Furthermore, men who eat, on average, 10.2 grams of cereal fibre a day are 30 per cent less likely to develop type 2 diabetes than those who eat 2.5 grams a day. Women who eat an average of 7.5 grams of cereal fibre a day are 28 per cent less likely to develop diabetes than women who eat 2 grams a day.[85] In other words, eating whole grains helps tackle some stroke risk factors.

Despite these benefits, 95 per cent of adults in the UK do not eat enough whole grains. Nearly a third do not eat any. The British Dietetic Association advocates getting at least half your starchy carbohydrates from whole grains (two to three servings daily). Try eating more foods with 'whole' in front of the grain's name – such as whole-wheat pasta and whole oats.

Seeds, nuts, legumes and pulses

Seeds, nuts and legumes are an excellent source of fibre and other nutrients. Peas, lentils, chickpeas and string beans contain up to twice the levels of vitamins and minerals as cereals, for example, and are rich in iron, zinc, selenium, magnesium, manganese, copper and nickel. However, plants use energy stored in seeds to aid the plant's early growth and development. So, they are relatively high in calories.

Not all 'nuts' are, strictly, nuts. Brazil and cashew nuts are seeds, for example. Peanuts are legumes, more closely related to peas and lentils than chestnuts and hazelnuts. You can ponder such botanical quibbles while eating a handful of almonds, cashews, walnuts, Brazils and pecans a day as snacks, while eating them with cereal and using them in baking.

Legumes and their seeds (pulses) are high in protein and fibre, and help control levels of fats in the blood. So, try to eat more:

- baked beans (although watch the sugar and salt in some brands);
- black beans;
- butter beans;
- chickpeas;
- haricot beans;
- kidney beans;
- mung beans;
- red and green lentils;
- soya beans; and
- split peas.

Eating one serving (130 grams) of pulses (beans, chickpeas, lentils or peas) a day lowers LDL cholesterol levels.[81] Vegetarian cookbooks are full of ideas to boost your bean, pulse and legume consumption. You can add these to 'bulk' up stews if you are cutting down on red meat, a leading source of saturated fat.

Watch the fat

As we have seen, high levels of LDL cholesterol in the blood increases the risk of stroke (see page 18). The risk is even higher in people who smoke or are inactive, the Stroke Association points out. However, the amount of cholesterol in your blood depends more on the saturated fat than the cholesterol you eat. Few foods – with the exceptions of eggs, kidneys, prawns and liver – contain high levels of cholesterol. As a result, diet accounts for only around a third of the cholesterol in our bodies.

As we shall see later in the chapter, eating enough protein reduces the risk of stroke by up to 20 per cent. However, you need to choose the right sort of protein. Fish reduces stroke risk. Red meat makes strokes more likely[78] and some cuts, especially fatty cuts and processed foods, contain large amounts of saturated fat. In other words, eating fish seems to reduce stroke risk, eating red meat seems to increase the risk.

Types of fat

Broadly, foods contain two types of fat:

- Saturated fat comes mainly from animal sources, and is solid at room temperature. For example, bacon rind, hard cheese and butter are high in saturated fats.
- Unsaturated fat derives mainly from vegetables, nuts and seeds, and is usually liquid at room temperature.

There are two main subtypes of unsaturated fat:

- monounsaturated (found in, for example, olive oils and avocados); and
- polyunsaturated (such as sunflower oil) – fish is especially high in a particularly beneficial polyunsaturated fat (see page 96).

Rather than worrying about the cholesterol in your diet, focus on the amount of saturated fat. The liver converts saturated fat into cholesterol. You can reduce the amount of fat you eat by choosing the leanest cuts of meat, trimming any visible fat and not eating chicken skin, pork crackling or bacon rind. Chicken, for example, has most of the fat outside the muscle, which you can easily remove. Currently, the British Dietetic Association notes, most people in the UK eat about 20 per cent more than the recommended levels of saturated fat (no more than 20 grams a day for women and 30 grams a day for men). Most of us should eat more low-fat foods, which contain 1.5 grams or less saturated fat per 100 grams. High-fat foods contain more than 5 grams of saturated fat per 100 grams.

Changing to a low-fat diet can be tough. But it's worth making the effort. If these changes do not reduce your blood cholesterol level sufficiently, you may need to take medicines. However, these are an addition to a low-fat diet. They are never a replacement.

Protein

Over the past 20 years, the evidence that dietary protein reduces stroke risk, in part at least by lowering blood pressure, has grown steadily. For instance, researchers looked at seven studies, which followed 254,489 people for 14 years. People with the highest protein intake were 20 per cent less likely to suffer a stroke than those who ate the least, after allowing for other risk factors. Each 20 grams per day increase in protein reduced the risk of stroke by 26 per cent. The benefit was especially marked against intracerebral haemorrhage: a 43 per cent reduction.[86]

In addition, protein helps you recover from a stroke by:

- helping repair and regenerate muscle, nerve cells and other tissues;
- forming specialized proteins, including enzymes that speed up the chemical reactions that are essential for life;
- building the scaffold that supports our cells' shape and divide the cell into compartments with specific roles; and
- making antibodies, which are essential for fighting infections.

The British Dietetic Association suggests that the 'general sedentary population' should eat between 0.80 and 1.0 grams of protein for each kilogram of bodyweight each day. Slightly more is needed by endurance athletes (1.2–1.4 grams per kilogram of bodyweight per day) and strength athletes (1.2–1.7 grams per kilogram of bodyweight per day). Your dietician will tell you if you need a protein-rich diet to help you recover from the stroke.

Fish and omega-3 fatty acids

Life inside the Arctic Circle is tough. As few plants survive, the traditional diet of First Nation Arctic people consists of fish and animals that, in turn, eat marine life, such as seals. Yet First Nation people who eat the traditional meat-based diet seem to be less likely to develop several diseases – including diabetes, heart disease, arthritis and asthma – than people in 'industrialized' countries. Furthermore, numerous studies show that eating fish protects against ischaemic stroke.[78]

Fish and, therefore, animals that survive on marine life are rich in omega-3 fatty acids, also called omega-3 polyunsaturated fatty acids (PUFA). These account for much of the benefit offered by the Arctic diet. For example, omega-3 PUFAs, among their other actions, reduce blood pressure, improve the profile of cholesterol and other fats in your blood and optimize platelet function (see page 55). These and other benefits help reduce the risk of stroke.[78] Omega-3 PUFAs are also important for memory, intellectual performance and healthy vision – all of which are commonly affected by a stroke. Eating oily fish, the British Dietetic Association points out, also keeps joints healthy. As rehabilitation can place extra stresses and strains on your joints, they are worth protecting, especially given the other actions of omega-3 PUFAs.

Humans can make omega-3 fatty acids from another fat (alpha-linolenic acid) in green leafy vegetables, nuts, seeds and their oils. But it is a slow process. So, eating fish (see Table 6.4) and seafood high in omega-3 PUFAs boosts levels of this essential nutrient.

The UK's national guidance for stroke suggests eating two portions of oily fish per week (salmon, trout, herring, pilchards, sardines or fresh tuna).[5] Omega-3 PUFA levels are higher in fresh fish. If you are eating canned fish, check the label to make sure processing has not depleted the omega-3 oils. I believe that it is worth trying to check that the fish comes from sustainable stocks (see <www.fishonline.org> and <www.greatdorsetseafood.org.uk/fishadviser>).

Table 6.4 Examples of fish and seafood high in omega-3 fatty acids

Anchovy

Black cod (sablefish)

Crab

Dogfish (rock salmon)

Halibut

Herring

Mackerel

Mussels

Oysters

Pilchards

Rainbow trout

Sardines

Salmon

Tuna (especially bluefin)

Adapted from the University of Michigan and the British Dietetic Association

If at first you do not like the taste of oily fish, do not give up without trying some different sources (see Table 6.4) and a few recipes. There are plenty of suggestions on the internet (for example, see <www.thefishsociety.co.uk>) and in cookbooks. For an island nation, our tastes in fish are remarkably conservative.

Exercise

Regular exercise is one of the best ways to avoid a stroke. The Stroke Association notes that even moderate exercise can reduce the risk of a stroke by up to 27 per cent. To look at the link another way: if you are physically inactive, you are 50 per cent more likely to suffer an ischaemic stroke than if you exercise regularly. Furthermore, exercise can boost levels of 'healthy' HDL cholesterol (see page 34), lower blood pressure and help prevent diabetes.[7]

Most survivors – about 80 per cent – resume walking in the year after the stroke. Yet despite its benefits, many survivors have problems getting enough exercise. Some worry about triggering another stroke. Indeed, two in every five survivors do not get out as much as they would like, partly because they worry about falling over and lack confidence.[3] If this sounds like you, speak to your doctor, physiotherapist or a patient group.

The UK's guidance for stroke suggests taking at least 2.5 hours of moderate-intensity exercise each week in bouts of at least 10 minutes. For example, you could go for a 30-minute walk five times a week. Stroke survivors should take part in activities that strengthen muscle activities and, if you are at risk of falls, that improve balance and co-ordination. In both cases, you should work out at least twice per week.[5]

The Stroke Association suggests starting gently – for example, a very short walk or a few minutes on an exercise bike or a slow treadmill. Then slowly increase the time you exercise for. However, check the exercise regimen with your GP or stroke team before starting. You should stop exercising and seek medical help immediately if you experience any of the following:[49]

- chest pain or angina;
- light-headedness;
- confusion;
- cold or clammy skin.

Make exercise part of your everyday life

You should try to make exercise part of your everyday life. If you exercise regularly for a year, you will lose about half your cardiovascular fitness in just three months if you stop. So, find a type of exercise that you enjoy and that fits into your lifestyle. If you do not like exercise classes and you join a gym some distance from home or work, you are more likely to quit. On the other hand, there are plenty of opportunities make exercise part of your day-to-day life:

- walk to the local shops instead of taking the car;
- ride a bike to work instead of travelling by car or public transport;
- park a 15-minute walk from your place of work;
- if you take the bus, Tube or metro, get off one or two stops early;
- use the stairs instead of the lift;
- clean the house regularly and wash your car by hand;
- grow your own vegetables – and they taste better;
- take your dog for more walks.

However, you need to dress for success. Make sure your footwear is appropriate. Your occupational therapist or physiotherapist can provide advice tailored to you. As a rule, most stroke survivors prefer training shoes, or flat supportive shoes with ankle support when walking. Loose clothes – such as jogging clothes – help ensure you have sufficient movement when exercising, even if you are just walking around the shops.[3]

Back to nature

You should also try to get out of town. Strolling around country parks and nature reserves brings benefits besides boosting fitness. In one study, people who had a view of a natural setting recovered from surgery more rapidly than a similar group who faced a wall.[87] Similarly, Japanese people with long-term illnesses often benefit from walking in woods – called *shinrin-yoku* (forest bathing). Scientific studies suggest that, among other benefits, *shinrin-yoku* encourages relaxation, reduces stress, lowers blood pressure and boosts the immune system. Even looking at, for example, a picture of people walking in a forest reduces blood pressure. However, the smell and other sensations of walking through a forest augment the visual appreciation of natural beauty.[88]

So, make the most of the more than 400 country parks and many other nature reserves in England alone. If you are worried about tripping and falling, call the reserve in advance or look for those with prepared paths (such as many National Trust properties). The following are good places to start:

- Natural England – <www.naturalengland.org.uk/ourwork/enjoying/places/countryparks/countryparksnetwork/findacountrypark>;
- The National Trust – <www.nationaltrust.org.uk/>;
- The Ramblers – <www.ramblers.org.uk/go-walking.aspx>;
- The Royal Society for the Protection of Birds – <www.rspb.org.uk/reserves>;
- The Woodland Trust – <visitwoods.org.uk>.

Smoking and drinking

Unless you have struggled with being hooked on a legal or illegal drug, it is easy to dismiss addiction, dependency and heavy use as lifestyle choices. Initially, people use legal and illegal drugs because they enhance enjoyment, take the edge off stress or help them cope with difficulties. However, addiction soon erodes the person's ability to say no. The compulsion overwhelms all their good intentions and lays siege to every intellectual, rational and emotional defence the user can muster, until he or she can no longer resist addiction's assault.

As we have seen, illicit drugs (such as amphetamines, cocaine and ecstasy) and legal drugs (such as tobacco and alcohol) can dramatically increase the likelihood of experiencing a stroke. In this section, we will look at some ways you can tackle abuse of legal drugs. If you need help with abuse of illegal drugs or legal highs follow the advice on page 41.

Drink to your health?

The rising tide of liver disease and the burden imposed by alcohol-related injuries on already stretched casualty departments illustrate the harm caused by excessive drinking. A quarter of admissions to intensive care units in Scotland in 2009 were alcohol-related, for instance.[89]

Nevertheless, many health problems emerge only after years of heavy drinking. For example, excessive alcohol consumption causes around one in every 25 cancers,[90] including those of the mouth and throat, oesophagus (food pipe), colon (large bowel), rectum, larynx (voice box), breast and liver.[91] Indeed, the liver, which breaks alcohol down, bears the brunt of the ill effects. Almost all men who usually drink more than 40–80 grams of alcohol a day (5 to 10 units) for between 10 and 12 years develop alcoholic liver disease. In women, drinking more than 20–40 grams a day (2.5 to 5 units) for 10 to 12 years makes alcoholic liver disease almost inevitable.[91]

Heavy drinkers do not just harm themselves. Alcohol abuse can irreversibly damage unborn children, destroy families or cause accidents that injure or kill others. If you know someone who is abusing alcohol you should – gently and sympathetically – advise them to seek help.

While there is conflicting evidence over the health benefits of light and moderate alcohol consumption, there is no doubt that heavy drinking increases risk of stroke. People who regularly consume large amounts of alcohol are three times more likely to suffer a stroke compared to teetotallers, the Stroke Association warns.

A UK unit of alcohol

A UK unit (see page 42) of alcohol contains 8 grams of alcohol. So:

- half a pint of normal-strength beer, lager or cider equals one unit;
- one small (100 millilitre) glass of wine equals one unit;
- a large (175 millilitre) glass of wine equals two units;
- a single (25 millilitre) measure of spirits equals one unit;
- one 275 millilitre bottle of alcopop (5.5 per cent volume) equals 1.5 units.

For example, researchers from Finland followed 2,609 men who had not suffered a stroke for, on average, about 20 years. During this time, 66 men died from stroke. Stroke accounted for about 2 per cent of deaths among men who drank, on average, less than once a fortnight rising to almost 5 per cent in men that drank five times a fortnight.[92]

In this study, after allowing for other factors that influence stroke risk – such as blood pressure, smoking, body mass index (BMI; see page 109) and diabetes – men who drank alcohol less than once every two weeks were 30 per cent less likely to die from stroke than non-drinkers. This supports suggestions that very light drinking may reduce the risk of cardiovascular disease. However, men who drank more than five times a fortnight were more than twice as likely (144 per cent increase) to die from stroke than teetotallers. The results were very similar when researchers took the total amount of alcohol consumed into account: men who consumed alcohol more than five times a fortnight were about three times more likely to die from stroke.[92]

Am I drinking excessively?

The NHS recommends not regularly drinking more than three to four units a day if you are a man or two to three units daily if you are a woman. If you have suffered a stroke or TIA or have another health problem, you should follow your doctor's advice: your limit may differ from the government's recommendation.

Doctors can use several questionnaires to detect alcohol abuse, including the CAGE questionnaire. You may have an alcohol problem if you answer 'yes' to two or more of these questions:

- C (cut) – Have you ever felt you should cut down on your drinking?
- A (annoyed) – Have people annoyed you by criticizing your drinking?
- G (guilty) – Have you ever felt bad or guilty about your drinking?
- E (eye opener) – Have you ever had a drink first thing in the morning to steady your nerves or to get rid of a hangover?

CAGE is not perfect. The 'ever' phrase means that the questionnaire captures people who had a drink problem but now abstain or drink safely. The Alcohol Use Disorders Identification Test (AUDIT) is a more detailed questionnaire (see <www.patient.co.uk/doctor/Alcohol-Use-Disorders-Identification-Test-(AUDIT).htm>). But don't leave it too late: most people deny that they abuse alcohol until they have to face health, social or legal problems.

Tips to cut down

Most people want to tackle problem drinking themselves before seeing a doctor or joining a support group such as Alcoholics Anonymous. The first step is to keep a diary of how much you drink and when (places and circumstances – such as when you are feeling down or stressed out) over a month or so. You need to note how much you drink and not just guess. According to Alcohol Concern, the average adult drinker underestimates consumption by the equivalent of a bottle of wine each week; a 750 millilitre bottle of wine that is 12 per cent alcohol by volume (ABV) contains nine units. You may find that keeping track means you start cutting down. If you get so drunk that you cannot recall how much you drank, you have a problem.

Your drinking pattern offers another clue. Most people vary their drinking pattern. People who abuse alcohol tend to drink more regularly, in some cases because they need to stave off withdrawal symptoms, such as the shakes, insomnia, agitation and depression. Returning to your old pattern after abstaining for a while is common among people who abuse alcohol.

You should set yourself a goal. But if you suffer from a serious disease speak to your doctor first. Some people who drink heavily will need to abstain, probably for the rest of their life. However, other people find that they can cut back and drink within the recommended limit – but they need to remain alert for changes in their drinking habits. It's all too easy to slip back into bad habits.

Some people pick a day and decide that they will stop or dramatically cut down. However, even if you plan to return to drinking safe levels of alcohol, it is worth 'drying out' and not drinking for at least a month to allow your body a chance to recover. (If you cannot stop drinking for a few weeks, you probably have an alcohol problem.) Other people find that it is easier to reduce the amount they drink gradually. So, it is important to keep using your diary to track your progress and help avoid any slips.

Simple tricks to cut back on drinking

Various tricks can help you reduce your consumption of alcohol:

- Replace large glasses with smaller ones.
- Use a measure to tell how many units of gin you are adding to your tonic or how many fingers of whisky you are pouring at home.
- Drink alcohol only with a meal.
- Look at the label and avoid wine with ABV of 14 per cent or 15 per cent. Try to buy bottles containing around 10 per cent ABV.
- Alternate alcoholic beverages with water or soft drinks. This reduces the amount of alcohol you drink and helps avoid dehydration.
- Mix your drink – try spritzers and shandies rather than plain wine and beer.
- Quench your thirst with a soft drink.
- Make sure you have 'dry' (drink-free) days each week. You may need to avoid your usual haunts and drinking partners on dry days. An environment that you associate with drinking can prompt you to have a drink.
- Find a hobby that does not involve drinking.
- Buying rounds can rapidly rack up the amount you consume. A group tends to keep pace with the fastest drinker. Try to buy rounds only for small groups.
- Ask for bottles of beer, shandies and spritzers, or halves instead of pints.

Whether to tell your family, friends and colleagues that you are trying to cut down on alcohol can be difficult. Some family and friends offer advice and support. Others may feel that you are challenging their drinking habits – and may prove hostile or condescending, especially if some of your social life or occupation revolves around drinking. In such cases, offer to be the designated driver or tell a white lie and claim that you're on medication and your doctor has advised you not to drink.

If you just cannot quit

Several books and websites can help you reduce your drinking. If you feel you really cannot quit without help, your doctor can refer you to NHS alcohol services or offer drugs to help you deal with cravings. Cognitive behavioural therapists (see page 122) and counsellors can help you understand why you drink. They can also offer suggestions to help you cut down and deal with any difficult situations. A doctor might be able to address any underlying problem that has contributed to your drinking. For instance:

- If you rely on a nightcap to get to sleep, try the tips on page 117.
- If you drink to cope with pain, your doctor can suggest alternative painkillers.
- Some people abuse alcohol because they are depressed or anxious or suffer from another psychiatric illness. Again, counselling and drugs (e.g. antidepressants or anxiolytics) may help.

Alcohol is such a part of most people's everyday life that it is easy to underestimate the harm that excessive drinking causes, the numbers of lives it damages, the pain it causes. Some diseases may mean you need to become teetotal. If not, you need to ensure you keep your consumption in check.

The healthy alternative

Instead of alcohol, drink plenty of water, fruit juice and so on. Dehydration is relatively common after a stroke, partly because of swallowing problems and partly because survivors often rely on other people to get them a drink. In other cases, the stroke may leave the survivor less sensitive to thirst.[3] However, even in otherwise healthy people, mild dehydration can cause a variety of unpleasant symptoms, including:[93,94,95]

- constipation;
- increased risk of DVT (see page 22);[3]

- reduced vigilance and concentration;
- poor memory;
- increased tension or anxiety;
- fatigue;
- headache.

Many of these are common symptoms among stroke survivors, which is one reason why it is so important to remain hydrated. You could be making matters worse.

The NHS notes that adults should drink 1.2 litres (six to eight glasses of water) each day to replace fluids they lose in urine, sweat and so on. If you feel thirsty for long periods, you are not drinking enough. Increase your intake during exercise or hot weather (or in a hot ward), if you feel lightheaded, pass dark-coloured urine or have not passed urine within six hours. If you regularly feel thirsty despite maintaining your fluid intake, you should see your doctor. Excessive thirst can be a symptom of diabetes.

Quit smoking

Nicotine, the addictive chemical in tobacco, and the plant's scientific name (*Nicotiana tabacum*) 'honour' Jean Nicot de Villemain (1530–1600), a French ambassador to Portugal. Villemain introduced tobacco to Parisian society when he returned from Lisbon in 1561. Smoking rapidly became fashionable.

However, concerns that smoking harmed health soon emerged. In 1604, James I of England (James VI of Scotland) described smoking as 'loathsome to the eye, hateful to the nose, harmful to the brain, and dangerous to the lungs'. The German physician Samuel Thomas von Sömmerring noted a link between pipe smoking and lip cancer in 1795.[96] We now know that in the UK during 2010 smoking caused:[97]

- 86 per cent of lung cancers;
- 65 per cent of cancers in the mouth, throat and oesophagus;
- 29 per cent of cancers in the pancreas, the organ that produces insulin (see page 39); and
- 22 per cent of stomach cancers.

Smoking's increasing social unacceptability – just look at the huddles of smokers outside offices, pubs and restaurants – is good news for our health. Nevertheless, about 10 million people in Great Britain still risk their lives by smoking. Around half of those who do not quit smoking die prematurely from their addiction.

If the benefits to your health are not enough to make you quit, think of the harm you are doing to your loved ones. Second-hand smoke contains more than 4,000 chemicals, including about 50 carcinogens (cancer-causing agents). This chemical cocktail increases the risk that people who inhale second-hand smoke will develop serious diseases, including cancer, heart disease, asthma and sudden infant death syndrome. For example, the risks that a woman who has never smoked will develop lung cancer and heart disease are 24 and 30 per cent greater, respectively, if she lives with a smoker than if she does not.

Quitting smoking dramatically reduces your stroke risk. As mentioned before, compared to people who do not smoke, smoking increases the likelihood of stroke by 83 per cent in women and by 67 per cent in men. Quitting makes a big difference. Women and men who have quit smoking are just 17 and 8 per cent more likely, respectively, to suffer a stroke than life-long non-smokers.[22]

Making quitting easier

On some measures, nicotine is more addictive than heroin or cocaine. As a result, fewer than one smoker in 30 quits each year and more than half of these relapse within a year, partly because of the intense withdrawal symptoms, which can leave you irritable, restless, anxious, sleepless and intensely craving a cigarette. These generally abate over about two weeks.

If you cannot tough it out, nicotine replacement therapy (NRT) 'tops up' levels in the blood, without exposing you to the other harmful chemicals. So, NRT can alleviate the withdrawal symptoms and increase your chances of quitting by between 50 and 100 per cent. You can chose from various types of NRT:

- Patches reduce withdrawal symptoms over a relatively long time, but start alleviating symptoms slowly. That's why you wear them for several hours.
- Nicotine chewing gum, lozenges, inhalers and nasal spray act more quickly.

Talk to your pharmacist or GP to find the right combination for you. Doctors can prescribe other treatments, such as bupropion and varenicline. While these offer a helping hand, you still need to be motivated to quit.

More recently, e-cigarettes have reached the market, although their exact role in helping people quit and whether they harm those around you (for example, by leaving nicotine deposits around the house) remains unclear. One study included adults who made at least one attempt to quit smoking during the 12 months before the study using e-cigarettes only, NRT only or no aid during their most recent attempt. People who used e-cigarettes were more likely to report abstinence (20 per cent) than those who tried NRT (10 per cent) or no aid (15 per cent).[98] Levels of carcinogens and toxic chemicals are low in e-cigarettes and no serious adverse events emerged in experimental studies.[98] Nevertheless, e-cigarettes deliver nicotine and are, therefore, still highly addictive, and they have not been available for long enough to ascertain their long-term risks and benefits. So, switching to e-cigarettes should be a step towards quitting. Furthermore, far fewer studies have assessed e-cigarettes than the other forms of NRT. So, you should discuss the best approach for you with a doctor or a GP.

Tips to help you quit

In addition to NRT or e-cigarettes, a few hints may make life easier:

- Set a quit date, when you will stop completely. Smokers are more likely to quit if they set a specific date rather than saying, for example, that they will give up sometime in the next two months.
- Quit abruptly. People who cut back the number of cigarettes they smoke usually inhale more deeply to get the same amount of nicotine. Nevertheless, cutting back seems to increase the likelihood that you will eventually quit. So, while reduction takes you a step towards kicking the habit, do not stop there.
- Plan ahead. For a couple of weeks before you quit, keep a diary of problems and situations that tempt you to light up, such as stress, coffee, meals, pubs or breaks at work. Understanding when and why you light up helps you find alternatives or avoid the trigger.
- Try to find something to take your mind off smoking. If you find yourself smoking when you get home in the evening, try a new

hobby or exercise. If you find car journeys boring without a ciga-rette, try an audio book, a music CD or radio play. Most people find that the craving usually only lasts a couple of minutes.

• Smoking is expensive. Keep a note of how much you save and spend at least some of it on something for yourself.

• Tackle stress. Try exercise, or take part in a hobby that you enjoy.

If you still cannot quit, ask your GP if your area offers NHS anti-smoking clinics, which offer advice, support and, when appropriate, NRT. You can obtain a free 'quit smoking' support pack from the NHS Smoking Helpline (tel: 0800 022 4332).

The power of hypnosis

Essentially, hypnosis is focused attention and concentration. Some hypnotists describe the process as similar to being 'so lost in a book or movie that it is easy to lose track of what is going on around you'.[99] However, doctors still do not understand fully how hypnotism works.

Nevertheless, there is no doubt that for some people hypnosis helps control pain, alleviate stress and change harmful habits such as abusing alcohol, comfort eating or smoking. Hypnosis can increase the chances of quitting smoking almost five-fold, for example.[99] And hypnosis is safe. You will not lose control: a hypnotist cannot make you do or say anything he or she wants. You will be able to come 'out' of hypnosis whenever you want.[99] Some people also find that self-hypnosis helps. Numerous DVDs, CDs and books help you create the 'focused attention' that underpins hypnosis. Contact the British Association of Medical Hypnosis for further information.

Dealing with setbacks

Nicotine is incredibly addictive and, not surprisingly, most smokers make three or four attempts to quit before they succeed.[100] Regard any relapse as a temporary setback, set another quit date and try again. It is also worth trying to identify why you relapsed. Were you stressed out? If so, why? Was smoking linked to a particular time, place or event? Once you know why you slipped you can develop strategies to stop the problem in the future. So, as the old health promotion advertisement suggests, 'Don't give up on giving up.'

Lose weight

Carrying even a few extra pounds can dramatically increase your chances of suffering a stroke. For example, being overweight increases the risk of an ischaemic stroke by 22 per cent, according to the Stroke Association. Being obese increases the risk 64 per cent. Indeed, overweight people are likely to have several stroke risk factors, including high levels of cholesterol, hypertension and diabetes. Being overweight also makes exercise harder.

Nevertheless, weight is not a very good guide to your risk of developing stroke and other diseases. Weighing 14 stone is fine if you are 6 foot 5 inches. But you'd be seriously obese if you weigh 14 stone and you're 5 foot 6 inches. BMI takes your height and weight into account and so offers a better indication of whether you are overweight. For an easy way to calculate your BMI, see <www.nhs.uk/Tools/Pages/Healthyweightcalculator.aspx>.

Try to keep your BMI between 18.5 and 24.9 kg/m^2. Below this and you are dangerously underweight. A BMI between 25.0 and 29.9 kg/m^2 suggests that you are overweight. You are probably obese if your BMI exceeds 30.0 kg/m^2. However, BMI may overestimate body fat in athletes, body builders and other muscular people (such as hod carriers). On the other hand, BMI may underestimate body fat in older persons and people who have lost muscle, which can happen after a stroke.

Doctors and gyms can use a monitor to check your body fat. However, not all fat is equal. Abdominal obesity damages your health

Table 6.5 Waist sizes linked to health risk

	Health at risk by waist size	Health at high risk by waist size
Men	Over 94 centimetres (37 inches)	Over 102 centimetres (40 inches)
Women	Over 80 centimetres (32 inches)	Over 88 centimetres (35 inches)
South Asian men		Over 90 centimetres (36 inches)
South Asian women		Over 80 centimetres (32 inches)

Adapted from the British Heart Foundation

more than fat elsewhere in your body, especially in people of South Asian descent, who are more likely to have a stroke than Caucasians. So, waist size can tell whether your health is at risk (see Table 6.5).

Tips to help you lose weight

Unfortunately, losing weight is not easy – whatever the latest fad diets would have you believe. After all, millions of years of evolution drive us to consume food in times of feast to help us survive times of famine. And you cannot stop eating as you can quit smoking or drinking alcohol. However, the following tips may help:

- Keep a food diary and record everything you eat and drink for a couple of weeks. It is often easy to see where you inadvertently pile on the extra calories: the odd biscuit here, the extra glass of wine or full-fat latte there. It soon adds up. A food diary can also help you see if you are eating fatty or high-salt food. Watch the sugar (see box).
- Set a realistic, specific target. Rather than saying that you want to lose weight, resolve to lose two stone (about 12.5 kilograms). Use the BMI to set your target weight. Cutting your intake by between 500 and 1,000 calories each day can reduce bodyweight (assuming your BMI is stable) by between 0.5 and 1.0 kilograms each week.[101] Steadily losing around a pound or two a week reduces your chances of putting it back on again. If you are recovering from a stroke, ask your dietician or stroke team what your ideal weight should be and when to start dieting. You may need extra calories in the early stages of rehabilitation.
- Think about how you tried to lose weight in the past. What techniques and diets worked? Which failed to make a difference or proved impossible to stick to? Did going to a support group help?
- Do not let a slip-up derail your diet. Try to identify why you indulged. What were the triggers? A particular occasion? With particular people? Do you comfort eat? Once you know why you slipped you are better placed to avoid the problem in the future.
- Begin your diet when you are at home over a weekend or a holiday and you do not have a celebration (such as Christmas or a birthday) planned. It is tougher changing your diet on a Monday morning or when you are away in a hotel faced with fat-laden food, caffeine-rich drinks and alcohol.
- If this fails, talk to your GP or pharmacist. Several medicines may help kick-start your weight loss.

Watch the sugar

Sugars are more diverse than the white powder you sprinkle in your coffee. Sucrose, glucose, dextrose, lactose (mainly found in milk), fructose (fruit sugar), maltose and corn syrup are all different types of sugars.[10] Sugars are a great source of energy. However, too many of us eat too much sugar. The World Health Organization (WHO) currently suggests that adults should get no more than 10 per cent of their calories from free sugars – such as sugar added to food and drink – as well as natural sugars in honey, syrups and fruit juice. At the time of writing, WHO suggesting cutting this to 5 per cent. That is about the same as 25 grams – about 6 teaspoons – or the amount of sugar in just one can of soft drink.

Get your flu jab

Every year, several thousand people die from flu, and strokes peak during the winter, partly because influenza is more common then than at other times of the year.[31]

That is why it is so important to get your flu jab. According to one study, the flu jab cuts stroke risk by 24 per cent. However, influenza vaccination did not affect the chances of having a TIA. The reduction was strongest with vaccinations early in the flu season: when administered between September and mid-November, vaccination reduces stroke risk by 26 per cent compared with 8 per cent from mid-November onwards.[31] So, get the jab as soon as you can each year. (The vaccine's composition changes annually to protect you from the current most common and dangerous forms of the virus.)

If you are in a vulnerable group (such as being older or having a serious illness) or caring for a high-risk person, your GP surgery should offer you a flu jab. You are in a vulnerable group if, for example:

- you have suffered a stroke or a TIA;
- you have a heart problem, such as chronic heart failure or you need regular treatment for angina or heart disease;
- you have a chest complaint or breathing difficulties;
- you have kidney disease;
- you have diabetes.

If you feel you should have the jab, but are not offered it, speak to your GP or practice nurse.

7

Life after a stroke

Strokes strike suddenly, and depending on the severity, you may be back from hospital within a few days or weeks.[7] This gives you and your family very little time to prepare for life after a stroke, which can turn your relationships and the household upside down. This chapter looks at some ways stroke survivors and their carers can live with the mental, physical and emotional problems that can follow a stroke. However, again, this is a general guide. Your rehabilitation team will offer you advice tailored to your problems and circumstances.

Make your home safe

Despite being a sanctuary, our homes can contain numerous dangers. We are used to making sure our children and grandchildren remain safe. However, we also need to keep stroke survivors safe.

Marilynn Larkin, for example, recounts the case of stroke survivor with agnosia – the inability to recognize objects, persons, sounds, shapes or smells. However, the senses are not impaired and a person with agnosia does not have marked memory problems. This stroke survivor tried to brush his teeth with a pencil and almost drank detergent thinking it was a soft drink. So, if there is any risk make sure potential hazards (including sharp objects and cleaning supplies) are out of harm's way.[10]

On the other hand, rehabilitation depends on getting people back to as normal a life as possible. Taking part in community activities is an important part of rehabilitation. As far as possible people should shop, take part in sports and leisure activities, visit places of worship, and stroke support and other groups. The regular review with your doctor or stroke rehabilitation team should include participation in these activities. You might also want to raise the subject, especially if you think there is an issue.

In other words, 'overprotective' carers are often counterproductive and even trigger resentment. This means that the survivor, the carers and the family may have to tread a fine line. Do not overestimate your or, if you are a carer, the survivors' abilities. If you as a carer feel – or the stroke survivor insists – that he or she can do a task, you should remain with the person and monitor the activity to be on the safe side. This is especially important if the task is potentially dangerous, such as cooking or ironing.[10]

Reducing the risk of falls

Some simple precautions can prevent falls (see page 78). While stroke survivors are especially vulnerable to falls and broken bones, many of these suggestions are sensible for older people generally. My grandmother – who had not had a stroke, but was slightly disabled – used to furniture walk. She used the side of the furniture, the wall, back of chairs and anything else that came in reach to get around our house and her flat. I used to worry she would tumble, especially if one the chairs moved unexpectedly. Stroke survivors often furniture walk. Try to avoid furniture walking and use mobility aids instead.

An occupational therapist, physiotherapist or social worker can suggest mobility aids (such as walking sticks or a wheelchair) and specialist equipment (including book holders, which allow the person to turn a page if they have the use of only one hand, card holders and needle threaders) that helps you maintain your independence. The therapist can also adapt your wheelchair to meet your needs better, such as providing elevated foot and leg rests if you have swollen extremities or a removable armrest to help you slide in to the chair.[10] Even 'simple' walking sticks need to be appropriate for your height and weight. Never buy a walking aid without specialist advice.

Therapists and social workers can suggest adaptations to your home that make getting around safer and easier. Ramps, handrails and grab bars all reduce the risk of falls. On the other hand, badly fitting or inappropriate footwear (see page 99), rushing and cognitive problems can increase the risk. For example, a person with cognitive problems may take unnecessary risks.

If you are buying carpet, get one with a short pile. People with a cane, walker or wheelchair can find longer piles difficult to move around on. Tuck extension cables and leads away and ensure there is good lighting inside and outside the house. Stick down loose carpets and mats, and try to limit clutter, which can be a distraction and a trip hazard.

Using a bathroom

An accessible bathroom can help people keep clean without asking for help, which bolsters their self-esteem. However, several simple adaptations can make a big difference:[8,10]

- Liquid soap or a washcloth pouch can be easier to handle than a bar.
- Putting sponge around the base of hairbrushes, toothbrushes and bottles helps with grip.
- Toothpaste pumps are often easier to use that a tube.
- Try electric razors rather than blades.
- Many people find long-handled sponges help them keep clean.
- A seat or bench in the shower or bath can help people who are experiencing problems with balance, perception or strength.
- A rubber mat or decals can prevent slipping. Some new baths now come with non-slip surfaces.

Dealing with mental issues

You and your carers will probably need to deal with mental issues that can follow in the wake of a stroke. For example, about 20 per cent of survivors experience memory loss six months after their stroke. Some people find that they cannot focus on the task in hand or sustain their attention for very long. Others seem less alert and mentally sluggish, and do not seem to engage. Poor attention can cause or contribute to fatigue, depression and problems living independently.[5]

We looked at some ways you can compensate for memory loss on page 70. In particular, a regular daily routine helps you to remember to take your medicines at the appropriate time, to exercise regularly and to practise the skills you need to regain as much independence as possible. A regular routine can help your carers as well. However, some stroke survivors may wander off and forget where they are. In some cases, an identification bracelet or pendant can reassure the family and the survivor.[10]

Making dressing easier

You can make dressing and undressing easier in several ways. For example:[10]

- Wear loose clothing that closes at the front.
- Wear trousers and skirts with elastic waistbands.
- Lay clothes out in the order you put them on.
- Get dressed and undressed while sitting. If the edge of the bed does not offer enough support, sit on a chair.
- Put clothes on to your weak or disabled arm or leg first. Undress in the same order.
- If needed, use a buttonhook. Button clothes from the bottom up.
- Try Velcro if buttons prove too fiddly.
- Bright prints and complex patterns can confuse people with visual or perceptual problems. Buy solid colours and simple designs instead.
- If needed, attach a metal key ring loop to zips. Do any buttons up before using the zip.
- Occupational therapists may be able to teach people to dress one-handed.

There is space here to look at only some common issues facing stroke survivors. The range of adaptations and aids is wide, diverse and growing. So, talk to your rehabilitation team – there is a remarkable amount of help available for stroke survivors with cognitive and other disabilities.

Living with fatigue

According to the Stroke Association, 10 per cent of survivors said they were always tired and 30 per cent said that they were sometimes tired two years after their stroke. Indeed, 50 per cent of survivors interviewed at least a year after their stroke said that fatigue was their main problem. In another study, half of the survivors reported experiencing fatigue since their stroke. Of these, 43 per cent said that they had not received the help they needed.[5]

Post-stroke fatigue is not like 'normal' tiredness. You may feel you lack the energy to take part in everyday activities – such as shopping, using the telephone or caring for yourself. You might not have the energy to participate in your exercises, therapy or rehabilitation. You may find that you need to rest every day or almost every day. However, rest may not improve the fatigue and trying to 'soldier on' just makes matters worse.

The severity of fatigue and its impact on everyday life varies from person to person and does not seem to depend on whether you had a mild, moderate or severe stroke. So, why is fatigue common after a stroke?

The Stroke Association notes that in the weeks and months after a stroke, your body is still healing, and rehabilitation can burn off a lot of energy. Indeed, recovering from any major illness can leave you feeling tired. You have probably also lost stamina and fitness because you have not been able to get around much after the stroke. Over the longer term, a disability can make walking and other 'normal' activities more tiring than before your stroke.

A range of other factors can exacerbate fatigue. For example:

- the stroke itself, although doctors do not understand why;
- depression and anxiety (see page 118);
- some medicines – including certain antihypertensives, antiepileptic drugs, painkillers and antidepressants – it is always worth checking with your doctor as there are often alternatives;
- insomnia and sleep disturbed by pain;
- breathing problems;
- eating problems and poor nutrition – for example, low levels of iron levels in the diet can lead to anaemia (low levels of red blood cells, which carry oxygen from the lung to your muscles and other tissues).

Good sleep hygiene (see box) and a regular bedtime routine may help. During the day, you should give yourself plenty of time and set realistic expectations. Do not try to do too much too soon. You need to learn to pace yourself and take breaks before and after activities. As the Stroke Association notes, even talking to friends, taking a car journey and eating can prove tiring. In addition, the improvement is likely to be gradual and your energy is likely to wax and wane. You could try keeping a diary of your activities each day, which will remind you of your progress and help you find the right balance of activity and rest.

If you are having a good day, stick to your plans. If you do too much too soon, you may feel exhausted for the next couple of days.

Nevertheless, gradually increasing the amount that you exercise may help reduce your levels of tiredness.[7]

Tips for a good night's sleep

You can take several steps to help you (and your carer) sleep better:

- Wind down or relax at the end of the day – do not go to bed while your mind is racing or pondering problems. Try not to take your troubles to bed with you. Brooding on problems makes them seem worse than they are, exacerbates stress, keeps you awake and, because you are tired in the morning, means you are less able to deal with your difficulties. Try to avoid heavy discussions before bed.
- Do not worry about anything you have forgotten to do. Get up and jot it down. (Keep a notepad by the bed if you find you do this commonly.) This should help you forget about the problem until the morning.
- Go to bed at the same time each night and set your alarm for the same time each morning, even at the weekends. This helps re-establish a regular sleep pattern.
- Avoid naps during the day.
- Avoid stimulants, such as caffeine and nicotine, for several hours before bed. Try hot milk or milky drinks instead.
- Do not drink too much fluid (even if non-alcoholic) just before bed as this can mean regular trips to the bathroom.
- Avoid alcohol. A nightcap can help you fall asleep, but as blood levels of alcohol fall, sleep becomes more fragmented and lighter. Therefore, you may wake repeatedly in the later part of the night.
- Do not eat a heavy meal before bedtime.
- Although regular exercise helps you sleep, exercising just before bed can disrupt sleep.
- Use the bed for sex and sleep only. Do not work or watch TV in bed.
- Make the bed and bedroom as comfortable as possible. Invest in a comfortable mattress, with enough bedclothes, and make sure the room is not too hot, too cold or too bright.
- If you cannot sleep, get up and do something else. Watch TV or read – nothing too stimulating – until you feel tired. Lying there worrying about not sleeping just keeps you awake.

Dealing with emotional and psychiatric problems

Surviving a stroke and coping with the life-changing consequences is often devastating for survivors, their partners and their families. Stroke survivors often worry about work, their finances and relationships. Not surprisingly, many lose confidence.[12]

Yet, emotional problems are more common than the disability alone can explain. American researchers, for instance, looked at two groups of people who did not have fully functional legs. In the first group, the disability followed a stroke. In the second group, the disability followed an orthopaedic problem, such as a hip fracture or arthritis. Almost half the stroke survivors had depression compared with about a fifth of those with orthopaedic problems. People who had a TIA are as likely to be depressed a year later as those who had a full-blown stroke.[102]

Cognitive and communication problems can make assessing depression difficult. However, the healthcare team needs to address the issue. (If you are a carer and suspect the survivor is depressed, it's worth raising the issue with the healthcare team.) A stroke survivor with depression is three times more likely to die in the 10 years after the stroke than a stroke survivor without depression.[102]

Stroke survivors potentially experience a wider range of psychological issues than depression alone. One study, for example, looked at 178 people who survived their first stroke. Patients experienced various emotions, including anger, helplessness, loss of emotional self-control, indifference and even euphoria.[103] (In the latter case, the brain damage may inhibit the control over inappropriate euphoria.) In addition, around 20 per cent of stroke survivors experience anxiety,[12] which may emerge several months after the stroke.[5] These changes seem, in part, to emerge after damage the parts of the brain that regulate emotions.

Tiredness and fatigue following a stroke can also trigger or exacerbate depression. Furthermore, depression is often a normal part of grief (see page 63) experienced by stroke survivors and their carers.[10] After all, a stroke offers a stark reminder of your mortality. Survivors may be disabled and will almost certainly need to make lifestyle changes. Many survivors are especially vulnerable to depression and anxiety when they are discharged from hospital. Being back at home highlights the extent of their disability.[3]

As mentioned before, the relationship between depression and stroke runs both ways. Depression increases the risk of suffering a stroke by about 34 per cent. Several factors probably contribute to this link. For example, depressed people are more likely to smoke, drink heavily, eat an unhealthy diet and be physically inactive than those without a low mood.[104]

Anxiety after a stroke

Anxiety evolved to warn of, and deal with, potential threats. The heightened alertness helps detect danger. The changes in our bodies prepare us to fight or escape.[105] However, many stroke survivors develop generalized anxiety disorder (GAD) – a condition in which they are abnormally sensitive to possible threats,[105] particularly regarding health, security and welfare.[3,106] People with GAD usually recognize that their fears are unrealistic, excessive and inappropriate.[107] Nevertheless, GAD still compromises work performance, relationships and leisure activities. If you can answer 'yes' to either of the following questions you may have GAD and should think about seeing your doctor:[108]

- During the past four weeks, have you been bothered by feeling worried, tense or anxious most of the time?
- Are you frequently tense and irritable, and do you frequently have trouble sleeping?

Stroke survivors may experience panic attacks during which they hyperventilate – manifestation of anxiety. They may even mistake hyperventilation for another stroke. Some survivors develop phobias (another type of anxiety) about objects and situations that they associate with the stroke or around social situations.

Finally, some stroke survivors develop post-traumatic stress disorder (PTSD).[3] Patients with PTSD often report flashbacks that emerge 'out of the blue' and vivid dreams and nightmares. Typically, they avoid places and people that evoke memories of the trauma (such as where they had the stroke), refuse to speak about their experiences and feel constantly on guard or emotionally numb.

Stroke, mania and lost self-control

Occasionally, stroke survivors develop mania, essentially an unreasonably elevated mood. People with mania seem hyperactive, speak rapidly, have grandiose and unrealistic ideas, cannot sleep, are easily distracted and lack judgement.[109] For example, a person with mania may embark on seemingly ridiculous investments or business schemes. Mania seems to arise when the stroke damages part of the brain involved in self-control.[10]

This loss of self-control can emerge in other ways. For instance, almost 60 per cent of stroke survivors may exhibit disinhibition: in other words, they do not follow the usual social rules and conventions about what they say or do. So, a disinhibited person may seem tactless, rude and offensive. About one stroke survivor in ten can become aggressive – which can be another form of disinhibition.[103] One stroke survivor with mania removed his clothes in front of visitors, urinated in the ward and indulged in sexually inappropriate behaviour towards the nurses. He came to view the ward as a concentration camp and the medical staff as guards.

Fortunately, a range of medicines and other treatments can effectively manage mania.[109] Carers should ask the stroke team for advice about responding to inappropriate, distressing or aggressive behaviour.

Do not underestimate depression

If you have never experienced depression, it is difficult to appreciate the devastation the condition can wrought over your life. The intensity of depression in stroke survivors tends to reflect the severity of the cognitive, motor and activity limitations. In turn, depression can exacerbate other problems, limit recovery and even increase mortality.[5] So, it's important to get help for depression, anxiety or any other psychiatric condition, whether these emerge before or after your stroke.

If symptoms markedly affect your daily life, the doctor may suggest antidepressants or drugs to alleviate anxiety (anxiolytics). While drugs can ease the symptoms, they do not resolve the underlying problem. But don't dismiss drugs out of hand. It is often difficult to tackle your problems when you are carrying the burden imposed by depression or anxiety. Medicines may offer a 'window of opportunity' to deal with any issues you face.

Unfortunately, diagnosing depression in people who have survived a stroke can prove difficult. Doctors may misdiagnose cognitive problems as depression and vice versa, for example.[5] For example, fatigue and apathy after a stroke can arise from several problems other than depression.[2] On the other hand, therapists can pick up depression when the person shows poor concentration or does not progress as expected during rehabilitation.

Setting goals and structuring time – being organized and having a daily schedule, for example – can help tackle the stress and depression that follow in the wake of a stroke for survivors and their carers. Goals and a routine give you a sense of purpose[10] and help you feel that you exert some control over the stroke, rather than the stroke controlling survivors and carers. Increased social activities, hobbies and taking more exercise (especially in the countryside) often alleviate depression.[7,88] Carers should not use phrases such as 'pull yourself together', 'cheer up' or 'things could be worse'. These expressions suggest that the carer does not appreciate how dreadful the survivor feels, and they can just make stress and depression worse.[10]

Depression and partners

Stroke survivors are about twice as likely to commit suicide as the rest of the population, which underlines the devastation that can trail in a stroke's wake. Young people, those who have more than one stroke and those who spend a short time in hospital are the most likely to kill themselves.[3] Most people who commit suicide have depression.

Tragically, depression can leave survivors unable to seek help. Depressed people can feel they are living at the bottom of a deep well: even if they can see the light, it seems faint and distant, and there is no way to climb out. A partner can encourage a depressed or anxious stroke survivor to seek help. However, remember that any ladder offered by you as partner, or by a doctor or counsellor, may seem rickety and unstable. You can help engender the confidence the stroke survivor needs to climb out. Emotional support shows that you care and so boosts your partner's feeling self-esteem, which can take a battering in the wake of a stroke.

Emotionalism after a stroke

Usually, crying and profound sadness are the most reliable indicators of depression among stroke survivors. However, crying or, less often, laughing inappropriately can be a sign that the stroke has damaged their brain's ability to express emotions (emotionalism) rather than being a sign of depression or mania.

About 20 per cent of people show emotionalism during the six months after a stroke.[5] These episodes tend to last up to several minutes and can be distressing and interfere with rehabilitation.[5,10] About 10 per cent of stroke survivors have long-term emotionalism.[5]

Distracting the person can help indicate whether a person has depression or emotionalism. Often people with emotionalism stop when you change the subject or call their name. This is not usually the case with depression. Once a doctor has diagnosed emotionalism, you could simply ignore the outburst.

Counselling and cognitive behavioural therapy

Sharing problems, asking for advice or a considering a different perspective often helps you overcome problems arising from stroke specifically or with life generally. Your stroke team, GP or occupational therapist can put you in touch with, for example, stroke clubs, counselling, relaxation programmes, exercise groups or alternative therapies. The Stroke Association can also provide details of support in your area.

Counsellors use a variety of 'talking therapies' to help you tackle your problems. For instance, cognitive behavioural therapy (CBT) identifies the feelings, thoughts and behaviours associated with your stroke or unhealthy lifestyle, such as addiction or alcohol abuse. The therapist will help you question those feelings, thoughts, behaviours and beliefs. You learn to replace unhelpful and unrealistic behaviours with approaches that actively address problems.

CBT can also use gradual exposure to feared situations or activities. As mentioned, survivors can develop phobias, including fears about leaving the home or fears around places and circumstances that they associate with a stroke. During CBT, the survivor spends increasing time in situations that they find stressful, such as travelling on public transport or visiting a shopping centre. Another element of CBT, called cognitive restructuring, replaces unhelpful and detrimental thoughts or anxieties with more positive thoughts. CBT usually uses explicit goals, often broken into manageable, short-term objectives and supported by regular 'homework'.

In some cases, tensions arise because of worries about money, especially in younger people (see page 28). However, tensions after a stroke in a family often have their roots in more than money alone. For example, a stroke, especially in relatively young people, can dramatically alter the dynamics of a family's relationships. In such cases, counselling and other forms of family support might help address the range of issues.[64] It is worth making sure that any counsellor you speak to is familiar with the problems and issues facing stroke survivors and their families.

Meditation

Cardiologist Herbert Benson from Harvard University in the USA successfully treated his hypertension (see page 30) in the late 1960s using meditation. Benson went on to become one of the world's leading authorities on mind–body medicine.[110]

Meditation brings millions of people – from all religious backgrounds – inner peace, relief from stress and improved health. Prayer (ask your spiritual counsellor if you need help) is a form of meditation, for example. Many people from diverse religious backgrounds value yoga, which aims to harmonize consciousness,

Think about your breathing

One of the first things a yoga, martial arts or meditation teacher will probably tell you is that you are not breathing correctly. Most of us breathe shallowly, using the upper parts of our lungs. Try putting one hand on your chest and the other on your abdomen. Then breathe normally. Most people find that the hand on their chest moves while the one on the abdomen remains relatively still. To fill your lungs fully, try to make the hand on your abdomen rise, while keeping the one on the chest as still as possible. Breathing deeply and slowly without gasping helps relaxation. If you feel stressed out, try breathing in deeply through your nose for the count of four; hold your breath for a count of seven; then breathe out for a count of eight. Repeat the cycle a dozen or so times.

mind, energy and body. (The Indian root of the word 'yoga' means 'to unite'.) Essentially, yoga focuses on achieving controlled, slow, deep breaths, while the poses (*asanas*) increase fitness, strength and flexibility. So, yoga helps maintain suppleness of both body and mind (some of the poses require considerable concentration). If you want to take up or continue yoga or tai chi (a Chinese martial art that is another form of moving meditation) after a stroke or TIA, speak to your doctor first. You should also let the teacher know about your stroke or TIA. Contact the British Wheel of Yoga or the Tai Chi Union for Great Britain for more information.

Getting back to work

Many of us count the days until Friday night – or the years until retirement. Yet employment (even if it is unpaid) can help recovery from a stroke, physically and mentally. For example, returning to work after a serious disease reduces the risk of depression – partly because it is a sign that you are on the road to recovery. Work can also boost self-esteem: for many people work is an important part of who they are and their social standing.[3]

Of course, work also helps financially for the quarter of stroke survivors who are less than 65 years of age.[3] However, estimates of the proportion of people who return to work after a stroke vary widely – from between 7 and 10 per cent to 78 per cent – partly depending on the definition of 'return to work'.[3,64] Not surprisingly, having relatively intact cognitive abilities and being able to walk increase the chances of returning to work.[2]

Yet many people who could work (even part-time and in voluntary roles) do not. (I do not support 'forcing' people who are sick or disabled back to work by attacking benefits. However, helping people back into employment can aid rehabilitation and help get life back to normal.) So, ask your doctor's advice about whether and when you can return to work.

You will need to talk to your employer and colleagues, and explain your issues, such as any disabilities or fatigue before you go back. Occasionally, an occupational therapist may need to assess the workplace and work with you to develop a plan that minimizes, for example, physical strain, fatigue and the effect of poor concentration. The occupational therapist can also ascertain whether adapting any equipment or work practices could help. Your GP can refer you to an occupational therapist.

Your employer will welcome you back. Few employers want to lose an experienced member of staff. However, do not overload yourself when you first go back. You may need to ease yourself back gently – such as beginning with alternate half-days at work and working on light or less challenging duties – and gradually build up over several weeks. Try not to multitask and focus on one thing at a time, which is good advice for everyone! You may also be able to use advances in IT, such as voice-activated software if you have problems typing, or changing the size of the type on the screen if you find the text hard to read. You might find some time management approaches advocated by management gurus – such as using lists to define your priorities – useful if you have trouble remembering everything. Again, many healthy people could benefit from these approaches.

Make sure you are aware of the support available under the Equality Act 2010. Vocational rehabilitation services often target younger people.[64] However, the access-to-work scheme helps people who are disabled or have a physical or mental health condition return to or stay in work, or start a business (see <www.gov.uk/access-to-work/overview>). A medical social worker may be able to help you access these support you need.

Driving after a stroke

Driving helps a stroke survivor get around and boosts self-esteem, self-confidence and mood. Driving, like getting back to work, is a tangible sign that life is getting back to normal. At the time of writing, you must not drive for one month after a single TIA or stroke, even if mild.

You can resume driving after a month if your doctor considers that your recovery is satisfactory. However, several factors may delay your return to driving, including experiencing more than one TIA 'over a short period', visual defects, seizures, cognitive defects and impaired limb function. In some cases, adaptations to the car may allow physically impaired stroke survivors to drive. Always consult your doctor and the Driver and Vehicle Licensing Agency (DVLA) or the Driver and Vehicle Agency (DVA) in Northern Ireland for advice before getting behind the wheel. If the doctor and DVLA or DVA agree, you must inform your insurance company.

Remember that even if you cannot return to your previous job, there are plenty of other opportunities, including the voluntary sector. Try to identify charities and non-governmental organizations that would benefit from your experience and that resonate with your interests and beliefs.

Sex and the stroke survivor

Stroke survivors and their partners often worry that sex could trigger another stroke or cause other problems. Occasionally, sex triggers an aneurysm to burst. So, people who have survived a haemorrhagic stroke should swallow any embarrassment and check with their doctor before having sex for the first time after the stroke. However, most stroke survivors can restart their sex life without worries. Sometimes a sex life even improves after a stroke: the increased opportunities to be close to, and intimate with, a partner increases sexual desire.[7]

Nevertheless, many stroke survivors do not feel sexually desirable. In some cases, physical changes makes them feel unattractive. In other cases, depression can cause erectile dysfunction or undermine libido.[10] However, never buy or use any treatment for impotence (whether bought 'over the counter' from a pharmacist or a herbal remedy) without speaking to your doctor. A male partner of a stroke survivor can also develop erectile dysfunction. For example, he may be afraid he will hurt his partner.[10] In other cases, a stroke survivor may not feel desire for a partner who has taken on more of a caring role.[10]

Talking to the stroke team, a counsellor or a patient support group often helps find a way around the problem. The Stoke Association also produces a range of helpful leaflets on sex after a stroke. You could try, for example:

- the partner taking a more active role if a physical weakness limits activity;
- taping a urinary catheter so that it does not get in the way.
- Problems with speech can undermine intimacy.[7] However, communication, especially in the bedroom, doesn't need to be verbal. And certain medications (including some antihypertensives, tranquillizers and antidepressants) may cause or contribute to erectile dysfunction, vaginal dryness and other sexual problems.[7,10] (A lack of a morning or overnight erection may be a

sign that the drugs are causing the problem.)[10] So, speak to your doctor. There is often an alternative drug or a way to compensate.

Stroke, your family and friends

As the effects on the sex life indicates, the relationship between survivors and their partners can change fundamentally. Some strokes reverse traditional gender roles. Spouses often shoulder considerable responsibility for implementing and supporting the lifestyle changes that reduce the risk of another stroke.[2] Your family can help you stay motivated when rehabilitation gets tough.

Even if you have problems talking, try to communicate with other people and not push them away. Communicating can help prevent isolation and loneliness. If you find communication difficult, you or your carer should ask your GP or stroke team for a referral to a speech and language therapist. A growing range of adaptations aid communication: think of Stephen Hawking's eloquence despite his profound disability.

Allowing your carer to help you helps your carer. Carers report better psychological well-being when they provide more assistance to the survivor. Interestingly, the severity of the survivor's physical disability does not influence the carer's psychological well-being.

Marriage can prevent stroke

Married people are less likely to develop several cardiovascular diseases than those who are single, divorced or widowed, researchers told the American College of Cardiology's 2014 meeting. They looked at the records of about 3.5 million people in the USA aged between 21 and 102 years. They allowed for other risk factors. Married people were 5 per cent less likely to have vascular disease than single people, and 9 per cent less likely to have cerebrovascular disease (affects the head's blood vessels). Widowers were 3 per cent more likely to have any vascular disease and 7 per cent more likely to have coronary heart disease. Similarly, divorce increased the risk of vascular disease, coronary heart disease and cerebrovascular disease. Marriage's benefits were especially marked in younger people. For those aged 50 years and younger, marriage reduced the risk of any vascular disease by 12 per cent, compared to 7 per cent for people aged 51–60 years and 4 per cent for those 61 years of age and older.

Carers – 70 per cent of whom are spouses – are less distressed when they care for a person who has survived a more severe stroke. This might be because people have higher expectations of recovery from a 'mild' stroke and the problems can be more subtle and frustrating.[111]

Holidays

A few days away helps you and your family relax. But plan carefully.

- Call ahead to make sure that the accommodation is suitable for your level of disability – such as allowing wheelchair access or not being at the top of a hill.
- Check that the accommodation is not too far from restaurants, shops and entertainment. (Google Maps with Street View may help.)
- Avoid places that are very hot or very cold. Your heart will have to work harder to keep your temperature at the right level. This places your cardiovascular system under more strain.
- Avoid high altitudes when travelling aboard. There is less oxygen in the air at high altitudes. Until you acclimatize (for example, by increasing production of red blood cells) your heart has to work harder, which places more strain on your cardiovascular system.
- Try to avoid stress – after all, a holiday is supposed to be a time to relax. You could return to a place you have visited recently to reduce the risk of unwelcome surprises.
- Leave plenty of time to reach the airport or destination.
- Do not carry heavy bags or rush around. People with health problems and disability may be able to get transport around the airport or ferry terminal, or port.
- Check with your GP or rehabilitation team (as well as the airline and travel insurance company) that it is safe to fly.
- Check that your travel insurance offers adequate coverage.
- Ensure you have information about local emergency and other health services in your destination – ask your tour operator. For holidays in the UK, you can check using NHS Choices.
- Check that you take sufficient medicines – a repeat prescription will not be available at the end of a phone call. Have a supply of your medicines in your hand luggage and in your suitcase, and take a list of all your drugs and doses. This is especially useful if

you visit an accident and emergency department or see an unfamiliar doctor.

- Make sure you check for any restrictions about bringing medicines (bought from a pharmacy or on prescription) into your destination. Some painkillers widely available in the UK are banned in certain countries, for example. You may want to check with the relevant consulate or embassy before you leave home.

A final word to carers

Caring for a stroke survivor can be tough. There will probably be times when the survivor does not seem to make progress or even appears to go backwards. So, remain as positive as you can and offer encouragement. However, avoid the temptation to do too much for the survivor. You need to walk a tightrope between helping and allowing the survivor to regain his or her independence and, therefore, self-esteem.

Some carers need to balance a job or childcare with looking after a stroke survivor, which can cause considerable stress. That might be one reason why older people caring for someone with a stroke are often more content than younger people.[111] They are more likely to be retired and less likely to have to juggle the responsibilities of a job and children alongside caring for the survivor.

Furthermore, your relationships can change fundamentally. Children or spouses may find themselves in a parental role. Stroke survivors may feel helpless and dependent – a bit like a child. The survivor may live overshadowed by stress and practical problems, be afraid of dying, and feel upset at not being able to take part in previously enjoyed activities. Not surprisingly, many survivors feel depressed, angry, guilty and bad-tempered, which can place a strain on your relationships. Involving survivors in decisions and conversations, even if there are problems understanding or communicating, underscores that they are still part of the family.[10]

Less obvious problems – such as cognitive problems, irritability, depression, fatigue and personality changes – tend to increase carers' stress and depression more than physical disability does. Dealing with incontinence as well as speech and communication problems can also prove especially stressful.[64] Indeed, carers report better psychological well-being – such as satisfaction with life, happiness and other positive emotions – when a survivor has fewer symptoms of depression.[111] This might be, in part, because many health services offer more resources for physical disabilities than problems with thinking, memory, behaviour and mood. Try to understand what the stroke survivor is going through – talk to the survivor, speak to patient organizations, and attend support meetings or stroke clubs. The Stroke Association offers family support services in some parts of the country.

In other words, living with a stroke survivor can be physically demanding, emotionally draining and highly disruptive. Not surprisingly, from time to time, carers feel frustrated, angry, resentful and even depressed. Other family members may feel they do not receive sufficient attention. Do not bottle these feelings up. Concealing or repressing your emotional pain and stress (or, indeed, a survivor bottling things up) can erode closeness in relationships. Talk about your feelings with your partner, friends and family, carers of other stroke survivors or a counsellor. Carers Direct is a national information, advice and support service for carers in England (see <www.nhs.uk/carersdirect>; tel: 0808 802 0202).

Carers report better psychological well-being when they are in better physical health.[111] So to look after your partner you need to look after yourself. Try to unwind while your partner is resting and get a good night's sleep – the tips on page 117 may help patients as well as carers. Do not feel guilty about taking time out for yourself. Carers who participate in the activities that they value feel they have greater control over their life, gain more from providing care and report better physical health and psychological well-being than those who give up activities that they once valued.[111]

A final word

Doctors, scientists and public health officials have made impressive progress tackling stroke over the last few years. Fewer people than a generation ago experience a stroke, the chances of surviving and making a full recovery are better than ever. Nevertheless, someone in the UK suffers a stroke every five minutes. One stroke in five is fatal. And despite the medical progress, you cannot rely on drugs and surgery to save your life. As Marilynn Larkin notes 'stroke happens in a moment but changes lives for ever'. But we have seen throughout this book that you and your carer can still live full and rich lives. I wish you both well.

Useful addresses

**Action on Smoking and Health
(ASH)**
Sixth Floor, Suites 59–63
New House
67–68 Hatton Garden
London EC1N 8JY
Tel.: 020 7404 0242
Website: www.ash.org.uk

Age UK
Tavis House
1–6 Tavistock Square
London WC1H 9NA
Helpline: 0800 169 6565
Website: www.ageuk.org.uk

Alcohol Concern
Suite B5, West Wing
New City Cloisters
196 Old Street
London EC1V 9FR
Tel.: 020 7566 9800
Website: www.alcoholconcern.org.
uk

Alcoholics Anonymous
PO Box 1
10 Toft Green
York YO1 7NJ
Helpline: 0845 769 7555
Website: www.alcoholics-
anonymous.org.uk

Atrial Fibrillation Association
PO Box 6219
Shipston-on-Stour
Warwickshire CV37 1NL
Helpline: 01789 867502
Website: www.atrialfibrillation.org.
uk

AVM Support (for people with
arteriovenous malformation)
Website: www.avmsupport.co.uk

Blood Pressure UK
Wolfson Institute
Charterhouse Square
London EC1M 6BQ
Tel.: 020 7882 6218
Website: www.bloodpressureuk.org

British Acupuncture Council
63 Jeddo Road
London W12 9HQ
Tel.: 020 8735 0400
Website: www.acupuncture.org.uk

**British Association for
Counselling & Psychotherapy
(BACP)**
BACP House
15 St John's Business Park
Lutterworth
Leics LE17 4HB
Tel.: 01455 883300
Website: www.bacp.co.uk

**British Association of Medical
Hypnosis**
45 Hyde Park Square
London W2 2JT
Website: www.bamh.org.uk

British Dietetic Association
Fifth Floor, Charles House
148/9 Great Charles Street
Queensway
Birmingham B3 3HT
Tel.: 0121 200 8080
Website: www.bda.uk.com

British Heart Foundation
Greater London House
180 Hampstead Road
London NW1 7AW
Tel.: 020 7554 0000 (general); 0300
330 3311 (helpline)
Website: www.bhf.org.uk

**British Medical Acupuncture
Society**
BMAS London
Royal London Hospital for
Integrated Medicine
60 Great Ormond Street
London WC1N 3HR
Tel.: 020 7713 9437
Website: www.medical-
acupuncture.co.uk
There is also a headquarters
covering the north of England,
sharing the same website:
BMAS House
3 Winnington Court
Northwich
Cheshire CW8 1AQ
Tel.: 01606 786782

Carers Trust
32–36 Loman Street
London SE1 0EH
Tel.: 0844 800 4361
Website: www.carers.org

Carers UK
20 Great Dover Street
London SE1 4LX
Tel.: 020 7378 4999
Website: www.carersuk.org

Chest Heart & Stroke Scotland
Third Floor, Rosebery House
9 Haymarket Terrace
Edinburgh EH12 5EZ
Tel.: 0131 225 6963 (general); 0808
801 0899 (helpline)
Website: www.chss.org.uk

Child Bereavement UK
Clare Charity Centre
Wycombe Road
Saunderton
Bucks HP14 4BF
Tel.: 01494 568900 (general);
0800 028 8840 (support and
information)
Website: www.childbereavement.
org.uk

**Complementary and Natural
Healthcare Council**
49 Queen Victoria Street
London EC4N 4SA
Tel.: 020 7653 1971
Website: www.cnhc.org.uk

Connect (for communication
difficulties)
St Alphege Hall
King's Bench Street
Southwark, London SE1 0QX
Tel.: 020 7367 0840; 01209 716501
(office in Cornwall)
Website: www.ukconnect.org

Cruse Bereavement Care
PO Box 800
Richmond
Surrey TW9 1RG
Tel.: 020 8939 9530 (admin); 0844
477 9400 (helpline)
Website: www.cruse.org.uk

Diabetes UK
Macleod House
10 Parkway
London NW1 7AA
Tel.: 020 7424 1000 (general); 0345
123 2399 (careline)
Website:www.diabetes.org.uk

Different Strokes (for younger stroke survivors)
9 Canon Harnett Court
Wolverton Mill
Milton Keynes MK12 5NF
Tel.: 01908 317618 or 0845 130 7172 (helplines)
Website: www.differentstrokes.co.uk

Disability Rights UK
Ground Floor CAN Mezzanine
49–51 East Road
London N1 6AH
Equality Advisory Support Service: 0808 800 0082
Independent Living Advice Line: 0300 555 1525
Website: www.disabilityrightsuk.org

Driver and Vehicle Licensing Agency (DVLA)
Vehicle Customer Services
Drivers Medical Enquiries
Swansea SA99 1TU
Tel.: 0300 790 6806
Website: https://www.gov.uk/government/organisations/driver-and-vehicle-licensing-agency

Driver and Vehicle Agency (DVA) (Northern Ireland)
Driver Licensing Division
County Hall
Castlerock Road
Coleraine BT51 3TB
Tel.: 0845 402 4000
Website: www.dvani.gov.uk

Focus On Stroke
For details about work on stroke being carried out by the NHS's National Institute for Health Research (NIHR)
Website: www.nocri.nihr.ac.uk

Heart UK – The Cholesterol Charity
Helpline: 0345 450 5988
Website: heartuk.org.uk

Independent Age (charity for older people)
6 Avonmore Road
London W14 8RL
Tel.: 020 7605 4200 (general); 0800 319 6789 (advice line)
Website: www.independentage.org

Institute for Complementary and Natural Medicine (and British Register of Complementary Practitioners)
Can-Mezzanine, 32–36 Loman Street
London SE1 0EH
Tel.: 020 7922 7980
Website: www.icnm.org.uk

InterAct Reading Service
Room 8, Victoria Charity Centre
11 Belgrave Road
London SW1V 1RB
Tel: 020 7931 6458
Website: www.interactreading.org

Internet Stroke Center
Website: www.strokecenter.org

National Osteoporosis Society
Camerton
Bath BA2 0PJ
Tel.: 01761 471771 (general); 0845 450 0230 (helpline)
Website: www.nos.org.uk

Northern Ireland Chest Heart and Stroke
21 Dublin Road
Belfast BT2 7HB
Tel.: 028 9032 0184
Website: www.nichs.org.uk

Rica (for mobility issues)
G03, The Wenlock
50–52 Wharf Road
London N1 7EU
Tel.: 020 7427 2460
Website: www.rica.org.uk

Royal National Institute of Blind People
105 Judd Street
London WC1H 9NE
Tel.: 020 7388 1266 (general); 0303 123 9999
Website: www.rnib.org.uk

Speakeasy (for aphasia)
1 Market Chambers
Ramsbottom
Bury BL0 9AJ
Tel: 01706 825 802
Website: www.buryspeakeasy.org.uk

Stroke Association
Stroke Association House
240 City Road
London EC1V 2PR
Tel.: 020 7566 0300 (office); 0303 303 3100 (helpline)
Website: www.stroke.org.uk

The Tai Chi Union for Great Britain
Media and Membership Officer
1 Littlemill Drive
Glasgow G53 7GF
Tel.: 0141 810 3482
Website: www.taichiunion.com

Vitalise (short breaks and holidays for people with physical disabilities and their carers)
212 Business Design Centre
52 Upper Street
London N1 0QH
Tel.: 0303 303 0145
Website: www.vitalise.org.uk

References

1 He F, Pombo-Rodrigues S, MacGregor G. Salt reduction in England from 2003 to 2011: its relationship to blood pressure, stroke and ischaemic heart disease mortality. *BMJ Open* 2014;4:e004549.

2 Good DC, Bettermann K, Reichwein RK. Stroke rehabilitation. *Continuum (Minneapolis, Minnesota)* 2011;17:545-67

3 Mant J, Walker M, editors. *ABC of Stroke*. London: BMJ Books, Wiley–Blackwell, 2011.

4 Mohan KM, Wolfe CD, Rudd AG, et al. Risk and cumulative risk of stroke recurrence: a systematic review and meta-analysis. *Stroke* 2011;42:1489-94.

5 Intercollegiate Stroke Working Party. *National Clinical Guideline for Stroke*. London: Royal College of Physicians, 2012. Available at: http://www.rcplondon.ac.uk/sites/default/files/national-clinical-guidelines-for-stroke-fourth-edition.pdf [accessed September 2014].

6 Souter C, Kinnear A, Kinnear M, et al. Optimisation of secondary prevention of stroke: a qualitative study of stroke patients' beliefs, concerns and difficulties with their medicines. *International Journal of Pharmacy Practice* 2014 [Epub ahead of print].

7 Lindley R. *Stroke: The facts*. Oxford University Press, 2008.

8 Hachinski V, Hachinski L. *Stroke: A guide to recovery and prevention*. London: Robinson, 2004.

9 Draaisma D. *Disturbances of the Mind*. Cambridge University Press, 2009

10 Larkin M. *When Someone You Love Has a Stroke*. New York: Dell Books, 1995.

11 Urban PP, Wolf T, Uebele M, et al. Occurence and clinical predictors of spasticity after ischemic stroke. *Stroke* 2010;41:2016-20.

12 Clarke DJ. The role of multidisciplinary team care in stroke rehabilitation. *Progress in Neurology and Psychiatry* 2013;17:5-8.

13 Hayes B. Delving into deep learning. *American Scientist* 2014;102:186-9.

14 Shipman P. Why is human childbirth so painful? *American Scientist* 2013;101:426-9.

15 Corbyn Z. Stroke: a growing global burden. *Nature* 2014;510:S2-3.

16 Bodak R, Malhotra P, Bernardi NF, et al. Reducing chronic visuo-spatial neglect following right hemisphere stroke through instrument playing. *Frontiers in Human Neuroscience* 2014;8:413.

17 Cresci G, Hummell AC, Raheem SA, et al. Nutrition intervention in the critically ill cardiothoracic patient. *Nutrition in Clinical Practice* 2012;27:323-34.

18 Greif DM, Eichmann A. Vascular biology: brain vessels squeezed to death. *Nature* 2014;508:50-1.

19 Bettex DA, Prêtre R, Chassot PG. Is our heart a well-designed pump? The heart along animal evolution. *European Heart Journal* 2014; 35: 2322–32.

20   Chambers T. *Stroke Care: Advancing practice in rehabilitation nursing.* Oxford: Blackwell Publishing Ltd, 2008:106-22.

21   Pound P, Bury M, Ebrahim S. From apoplexy to stroke. *Age and Ageing* 1997;26:331-7.

22   Peters SA, Huxley RR, Woodward M. Smoking as a risk factor for stroke in women compared with men: a systematic review and meta-analysis of 81 cohorts, including 3,980,359 individuals and 42,401 strokes. *Stroke* 2013;44:2821-8.

23   Matthews D, Beatty S, Dyson P, et al. *Diabetes: The facts.* Oxford University Press, 2008: 132-4.

24   The Internet Stroke Center. The ischemic penumbra. Available at: <www.strokecenter.org/professionals/brain-anatomy/cellular-injury-during-ischemia/the-ischemic-penumbra> [accessed September 2014].

25   Pettigrew LC, Dobbs MR. Stroke: thrombolysis and antithrombotic therapy. In: Moliterno DJ, Kristensen SK, de Caterina R, editors. *Therapeutic Advances in Thrombosis.* Oxford: Blackwell Publishing Ltd, 2012:272-84.

26   Kumar S, Selim MH, Caplan LR. Medical complications after stroke. *Lancet Neurology* 2010;9:105-18.

27   Faraco G, Iadecola C. Hypertension: a harbinger of stroke and dementia. *Hypertension* 2013;62:810-17.

28   Veillon EW, Martin JN. Pregnancy-related stroke. In: Belfort MA, Saade G, Foley MR, et al., editors. *Critical Care Obstetrics.* Chichester: Wiley–Blackwell, 2010:235-55.

29   Korja M, Lehto H, Juvela S. Lifelong rupture risk of intracranial aneurysms depends on risk factors: a prospective Finnish cohort study. *Stroke* 2014; 35:1958-63.

30   Synhaeve NE, Arntz RM, Maaijwee NAM, et al. Poor long-term functional outcome after stroke among adults aged 18 to 50 years: follow-up of transient ischemic attack and stroke patients and unelucidated risk factor evaluation (FUTURE) study. *Stroke* 2014; 45:1157-60.

31   Siriwardena AN, Asghar Z, Coupland CC. Influenza and pneumococcal vaccination and risk of stroke or transient ischaemic attack – matched case control study. *Vaccine* 2014;32:1354-61.

32   Huang Y, Cai X, Li Y. Prehypertension and the risk of stroke: a meta-analysis. *Neurology* 2014;82:1153-61.

33   Onusko E. Diagnosing secondary hypertension. *American Family Physician* 2003;67:67-74.

34   Viera AJ, Hinderliter AL. Evaluation and management of the patient with difficult-to-control or resistant hypertension. *American Family Physician* 2009;79:863-9.

35   Yamazaki T, Miyazaki M, Kanase H, et al. Transient hypertension in male adolescents when measured by a woman. *Heart* 1998;79:104-5.

36   Mulder BJ, van der Wall EE. Size and function of the atria. *International Journal of Cardiovascular Imaging* 2008;24:713-16.

37   Benjamin EJ, Chen PS, Bild DE, et al. Prevention of atrial fibrillation: report from a national heart, lung, and blood institute workshop. *Circulation* 2009;119:606-18.

38 Menaa F. Stroke in sickle cell anemia patients: a need for multidisciplinary approaches. *Atherosclerosis* 2013;229:496-503.

39 Ronksley PE, Brien SE, Turner BJ, et al. Association of alcohol consumption with selected cardiovascular disease outcomes: a systematic review and meta-analysis. *BMJ* 2011;342:d671.

40 Carey IM, Shah SM, DeWilde S, et al. Increased risk of acute cardiovascular events after partner bereavement: a matched cohort study. *JAMA Internal Medicine* 2014;174:598-605.

41 Mostofsky E, Penner EA, Mittleman MA. Outbursts of anger as a trigger of acute cardiovascular events: a systematic review and meta-analysis. *European Heart Journal* 2014;35:1404-10.

42 Breuer J, Pacou M, Gauthier A, et al. Herpes zoster as a risk factor for stroke and TIA: a retrospective cohort study in the UK. *Neurology* 2014;82:206-12.

43 Langan SM, Minassian C, Smeeth L, et al. Risk of stroke following herpes zoster: a self-controlled case-series study. *Clinical Infectious Diseases* 2014;58:1497-503.

44 Peragallo Urrutia R, Coeytaux RR, McBroom AJ, et al. Risk of acute thromboembolic events with oral contraceptive use: a systematic review and meta-analysis. *Obstetrics and Gynecology* 2013;122:380-9.

45 Siberstein S. A perspective on the migraine mind. *American Scientist* 2014;102:226-9.

46 Kurth T, Gaziano J, Cook NR, et al. Migraine and risk of cardiovascular disease in women. *JAMA* 2006;296:283-91.

47 Wagstaff AJ, Overvad TF, Lip GYH, et al. Is female sex a risk factor for stroke and thromboembolism in patients with atrial fibrillation? A systematic review and meta-analysis. *QJM* 2014 [Epub ahead of print].

48 Haslam F. *From Hogarth to Rowlandson: Medicine in art in eighteenth-century Britain.* Liverpool University Press, 1996:270.

49 Kilbride C, Kneafsey R. Management of Physical Impairments Post-Stroke. *Acute Stroke Nursing.* Oxford: Wiley-Blackwell, 2010:152-83.

50 Meretoja A, Keshtkaran M, Saver J, et al. Stroke thrombolysis: save a minute, save a day. *Stroke* 2014;45:1053-1058.

51 Yong E. First response: race against time. *Nature* 2014;510:S5.

52 Dennis M, Sandercock P, Reid J, et al. Effectiveness of intermittent pneumatic compression in reduction of risk of deep vein thrombosis in patients who have had a stroke (CLOTS 3): a multicentre randomised controlled trial. *Lancet* 2013;382:516-24.

53 Li J. *Block-buster Drugs: The rise and decline of the pharmaceutical industry.* Oxford University Press, 2014.

54 PROGRESS Collaborative Group. Randomised trial of a perindopril-based blood-pressure-lowering regimen among 6105 individuals with previous stroke or transient ischaemic attack. *Lancet* 2001;358:1033-41.

55 Law M, Wald N, Morris J. Lowering blood pressure to prevent myocardial infarction and stroke: a new preventive strategy. *Health Technology Assessment* 2003;7:106.

56 Neal B, MacMahon S, Chapman N, Blood Pressure Lowering Treatment Trialists' Collaboration. Effects of ACE inhibitors, calcium antagonists,

and other blood-pressure-lowering drugs: results of prospectively designed overviews of randomised trials. *Lancet* 2000;356:1955-64.

57   Williams B, Poulter NR, Brown MJ, et al. Guidelines for management of hypertension: report of the fourth working party of the British Hypertension Society, 2004 – BHS IV. *Journal of Human Hypertension* 2004;18:139-85.

58   Gradman AH. Rationale for triple-combination therapy for management of high blood pressure. *The Journal of Clinical Hypertension* 2010;12:869-78.

59   Pedersen TR, Kjekshus J, Berg K, et al. Randomised trial of cholesterol lowering in 4444 patients with coronary heart disease: the Scandinavian Simvastatin Survival Study (4S). *Lancet* 1994;344:1383-9.

60   Stamou SC, Hill PC, Dangas G, et al. Stroke after coronary artery bypass: incidence, predictors, and clinical outcome. *Stroke* 2001;32:1508-13.

61   Addington-Hall J. Heart disease and stroke: Lessons from cancer care. In: Ford G, Lewin IG, editors. *Managing Terminal Illness*. London: Royal College of Physicians, 1996.

62   Mueller P, Plevak D, Rummans T. Religious involvement, spirituality, and medicine: implications for clinical practice. *Mayo Clinic Proceedings* 2001;76:1225-35.

63   Dugan D. Laughter and tears: best medicine for stress. *Nursing Forum* 1989;24:18–26.

64   Brereton L, Manthorpe J. Longer-term support for survivors and supporters. In: Williams J, Perry L, Watkins C, editors. *Acute Stroke Nursing*. Oxford: Wiley-Blackwell, 2010:309-30.

65   Makin SD, Turpin S, Dennis MS, et al. Cognitive impairment after lacunar stroke: systematic review and meta-analysis of incidence, prevalence and comparison with other stroke subtypes. *Journal of Neurology, Neurosurgery and Psychiatry* 2013;84:893-900.

66   King K. *Ventriloquism Made Easy*. London: Dover Books, 1997:10-11.

67   Rofes L, Vilardell N, Clavé P. Post-stroke dysphagia: progress at last. *Neurogastroenterology and Motility* 2013;25:278-82.

68   O'Mahony D, O'Leary P, Quigley EM. Aging and intestinal motility: a review of factors that affect intestinal motility in the aged. *Drugs and Aging* 2002;19:515-27.

69   Diamant NE. Functional anatomy and physiology of swallowing and esophageal motility. In: Richter J, Castell DO, editors. *The Esophagus*. Oxford: Wiley-Blackwell, 2012:63-96.

70   Cichero JY, Steele C, Duivestein J, et al. The need for international terminology and definitions for texture-modified foods and thickened liquids used in dysphagia management: foundations of a global initiative. *Current Physical Medicine and Rehabilitation Reports* 2013;1:280-91.

71   Bansil S, Prakash N, Kaye J, et al. Movement disorders after stroke in adults: a review. *Tremor and Other Hyperkinetic Movements* 2012;2: pii: tre-02-42-195-1.

72   Costandi M. Rehabilitation: machine recovery. *Nature* 2014;510:S8-9.

73   Thibaut A, Chatelle C, Ziegler E, et al. Spasticity after stroke: physiology, assessment and treatment. *Brain Injury* 2013;27:1093-105.

74 Grunda T, Marsalek P, Sykorova P. Homonymous hemianopia and related visual defects: restoration of vision after a stroke. *Acta Neurobiologiae Experimentalis* 2013;73:237-49.

75 Vickers AJ, Cronin AM, Maschino AC, et al. Acupuncture for chronic pain: individual patient data meta-analysis. *Archives of Internal Medicine* 2012;172:1444-53.

76 Hao J, Hao L. Review of clinical applications of scalp acupuncture for paralysis: an excerpt from Chinese scalp acupuncture. *Global Advances in Health and Medicine* 2012;1:102-21.

77 Raghunathan S, Richard B, Khanna P. Causes and clinical characteristics of headache in ischaemic stroke. *Progress in Neurology and Psychiatry* 2008;12:21-3.

78 Tamayo A, Castilla-Guerra L. Dietary protein and stroke prevention: is the Eskimo diet the answer to avoid stroke? *Neurology* 2014;83:13-14.

79 Leach E. *Lévi-Strauss*. New York: Fontana, 1970:32-4.

80 Aliani M, Udenigwe CC, Girgih AT, et al. Aroma and taste perceptions with Alzheimer disease and stroke. *Critical Reviews in Food Science and Nutrition* 2012;53:760-9.

81 Hu D, Huang J, Wang Y, et al. Fruits and vegetables consumption and risk of stroke: a meta-analysis of prospective cohort studies. *Stroke* 2014;45:1613-19.

82 Oyebode O, Gordon-Dseagu V, Walker A, et al. Fruit and vegetable consumption and all-cause, cancer and CVD mortality: analysis of Health Survey for England data. *Journal of Epidemiology and Community Health* 2014;68:856-62.

83 Aaron KJ, Sanders PW. Role of dietary salt and potassium intake in cardiovascular health and disease: a review of the evidence. *Mayo Clinic Proceedings* 2013;88:987-95.

84 Yokoyama Y, Nishimura K, Barnard ND, et al. Vegetarian diets and blood pressure: a meta-analysis. *JAMA Internal Medicine* 2014;174:577-87.

85 Anderson JW, Conley SB. Whole grains and diabetes. In: Marquart L, Jacobs DR, McIntosh GH, et al., editors. *Whole Grains and Health*. Ames, IN: Blackwell Publishing Professional, 2007:29-46.

86 Zhang Z, Xu G, Yang F, et al. Quantitative analysis of dietary protein intake and stroke risk. *Neurology* 2014; 83:19-25.

87 Vallance AK. Something out of nothing: the placebo effect. *Advances in Psychiatric Treatment* 2006;12:287-96.

88 Tsunetsugu Y, Park B-J, Miyazaki Y. Trends in research related to "Shinrin-yoku" (taking in the forest atmosphere or forest bathing) in Japan. *Environmental Health and Preventive Medicine* 2010;15:27-37.

89 Geary T, O'Brien P, Ramsay S, et al. A national service evaluation of the impact of alcohol on admissions to Scottish intensive care units. *Anaesthesia* 2012;67:1132-7.

90 Parkin DM. Cancers attributable to consumption of alcohol in the UK in 2010. *British Journal of Cancer* 2011;105 suppl 2:S14-18.

91 Gramenzi A, Caputo F, Biselli M, et al. Review article: alcoholic liver disease – pathophysiological aspects and risk factors. *Alimentary Pharmacology and Therapeutics* 2006;24:1151-61.

92   Rantakömi SH, Kurl S, Sivenius J, et al. The frequency of alcohol consumption is associated with the stroke mortality. *Acta Neurologica Scandinavica* 2014;130:118-24.

93   Armstrong LE, Ganio MS, Casa DJ, et al. Mild dehydration affects mood in healthy young women. *The Journal of Nutrition* 2012;142:382-8.

94   Ganio MS, Armstrong LE, Casa DJ, et al. Mild dehydration impairs cognitive performance and mood of men. *The British Journal of Nutrition* 2011;106:1535-43.

95   Spigt M, Weerkamp N, Troost J, et al. A randomized trial on the effects of regular water intake in patients with recurrent headaches. *Family Practice* 2012;29:370-5.

96   Hajdu SI. A note from history: landmarks in history of cancer, part 3. *Cancer* 2012;118:1155-68.

97   Parkin DM. Tobacco-attributable cancer burden in the UK in 2010. *British Journal of Cancer* 2011;105 suppl 2:S6-13.

98   Brown J, Beard E, Kotz D, et al. Real-world effectiveness of e-cigarettes when used to aid smoking cessation: a cross-sectional population study. *Addiction* 2014:109:1531-40.

99   Montgomery GH, Schnur JB, Kravits K. Hypnosis for cancer care: over 200 years young. *CA: A Cancer Journal for Clinicians* 2013;63:31-44.

100 Russell A. *The Social Basis of Medicine.* Chichester: Wiley-Blackwell, 2009.

101 Toeller M. Lifestyle issues: diet. In: Holt RI, Cockram C, Flyvbjerg A, editors. *Textbook of Diabetes.* Chichester: Wiley-Blackwell, 2010:346-57.

102 Gupta S. Mental health: ups and downs. *Nature* 2014;510:S10-11.

103 Huang HC, Huang LK, Hu CJ, et al. The mediating effect of psychological distress on functional dependence in stroke patients. *Journal of Clinical Nursing* 2014 [Epub ahead of print].

104 Penninx BW, Milaneschi Y, Lamers F, et al. Understanding the somatic consequences of depression: biological mechanisms and the role of depression symptom profile. *BMC Medicine* 2013;11:129.

105 Bateson M, Brilot B, Nettle D. Anxiety: an evolutionary approach. *Canadian Journal of Psychiatry* 2011;56:707-15.

106 Allgulander C. Generalized anxiety disorder: a review of recent findings. *Journal of Experimental and Clinical Medicine* 2012;4:88-91.

107 Gale C, Davidson O. Generalised anxiety disorder. *BMJ* 2007;334:579-81.

108 Hoge EA, Ivkovic A, Fricchione GL. Generalized anxiety disorder: diagnosis and treatment. *BMJ* 2012;345.

109 Routh R, Hill A. Post-stroke mania: a rare but treatable presentation. *Progress in Neurology and Psychiatry* 2014;18:24-5.

110 Ausubel K. *When Healing Becomes a Crime.* Rochester, Vermont: Healing Arts Press, 2000;217, 351.

111 Cameron JI, Stewart DE, Streiner DL, et al. What makes family caregivers happy during the first 2 years post stroke? *Stroke* 2014;45:1084-9.

Further reading

Draaisma, Douwe. *Disturbances of the Mind*. Cambridge University Press, 2009.

Greener, Mark. *The Heart Attack Survival Guide*. London: Sheldon Press, 2012.

Greener, Mark. *The Holistic Health Handbook*. London: Sheldon Press, 2013.

Greener, Mark and Christine Craggs-Hinton. *The Diabetes Healing Diet,* London: Sheldon Press, 2012.

Hachinski, Vladimir and Larissa Hachinski. *Stroke: A guide to recovery and prevention*. London: Robinson, 2004.

Harrington, Anne. *The Cure Within: A history of mind–body medicine*. New York: W. W. Norton, 2008.

Larkin, Marilynn. *When Someone You Love Has a Stroke*. New York: Dell Books, 1995.

Lindley, Richard. *Stroke: The facts*. Oxford University Press, 2008.

Matthews, David, Sue Beatty, Pam Dyson, Laurie King and Aparna Pal. *Diabetes: The facts*, first edition. Oxford University Press, 2008.

Mant, Jonathan and Marion F. Walker (editors). *ABC of Stroke*. London: BMJ Books/London and Chichester: Wiley–Blackwell, 2011.

Russell, Andrew. *The Social Basis of Medicine*. Chichester: Wiley–Blackwell, 2009.

Sacks, Oliver. *The Man Who Mistook His Wife for a Hat*. London: Picador, 1986.

Index

If you are looking for the warning signs of a stroke please see pages ix and 15. If you or anyone else has any of these signs call for an ambulance immediately.